This book belongs to:

____

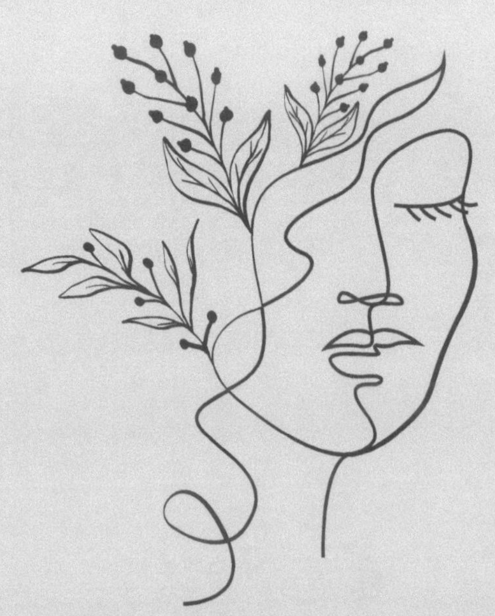

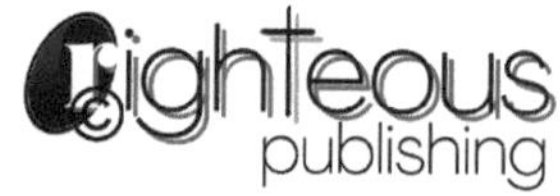

TEN WAYS YOU CAN COPE

TABLE OF CONTENTS

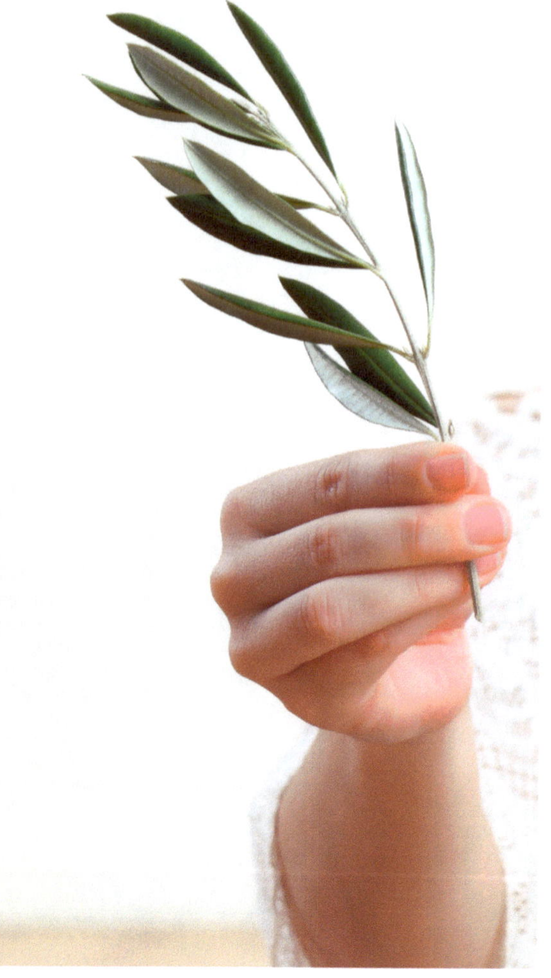

A NOTE FROM THE AUTHOR

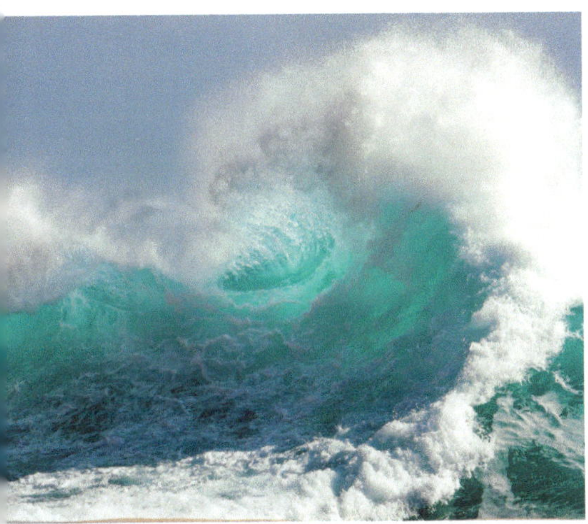

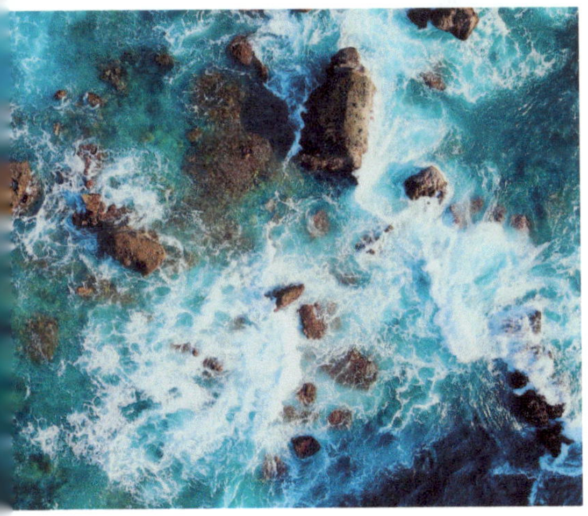

GET BACK IN

Have you spent any time in the ocean? One minute you're floating along minding your own business, and the next- you're spinning around uncontrollably. You can't breathe, you don't know which way is up, and you're not sure you're going to survive this. Sometimes you get slammed against the sand, which steals whatever breath you had left. It can be pretty scary.

But for some reason we go back in.

Life is like that. One minute we're enjoying our ever day life; working, playing, living, and the next we are completely overwhelmed. We can't breathe, we don't know which way is up, and we don't know how we will survive this. And oftentimes, life adds a little extra painful situation to what we were already dealing with- that good old slam into the sand.

When his happens, we can have a hard time shaking it off. The bruises last a long time, that pain lingers, but we can't just quit. We need to find a way to get through it. To feel it, heal it, and get back in the water.

My hope is that these ideas will help you do just that.

Charlaine

introduction...

HOW TO USE THIS BOOK

The truth is, you can use this book in any way you want. My hope is to **empower you** by offering some **simple coping skills**, and to **encourage you** to try them out. Sometimes the smallest things can make the biggest difference.

I'll offer explanations of ten ideas, and some examples of how you can practice them. I'll give you the chance to think of your own ideas, decide which one/s you'd like to try, and then I'll ask you to reflect on how well they worked for you.

You can do some or all of them. You can try them in the order I present them, or try the one that sounds most achievable to you right now. There is no wrong way to try.

Some things take practice, some will bring immediate gratification.

We cannot control much of this crazy world, but we can build confidence in our ability to handle whatever comes our way.

I believe in you. Let's learn to cope.

.

ONE: BREATHE

"Only those who know how to breathe will survive."
– Pundit Acharya

I have this habit of not breathing. Often I don't notice until I start feeling woozy or lightheaded. When I start to breathe again, I start feeling better. It's amazing how that works, it's like we're supposed to be breathing all the time. Duh.

Covid-19 brought with it mandatory masks, and if you have breathing issues, these masks likely heightened them. Sometimes it feels like you just cannot breathe at all, and that you are not getting the oxygen you need. Sometimes those masks feel so restrictive- in more ways than one. But we did our best. We tried.

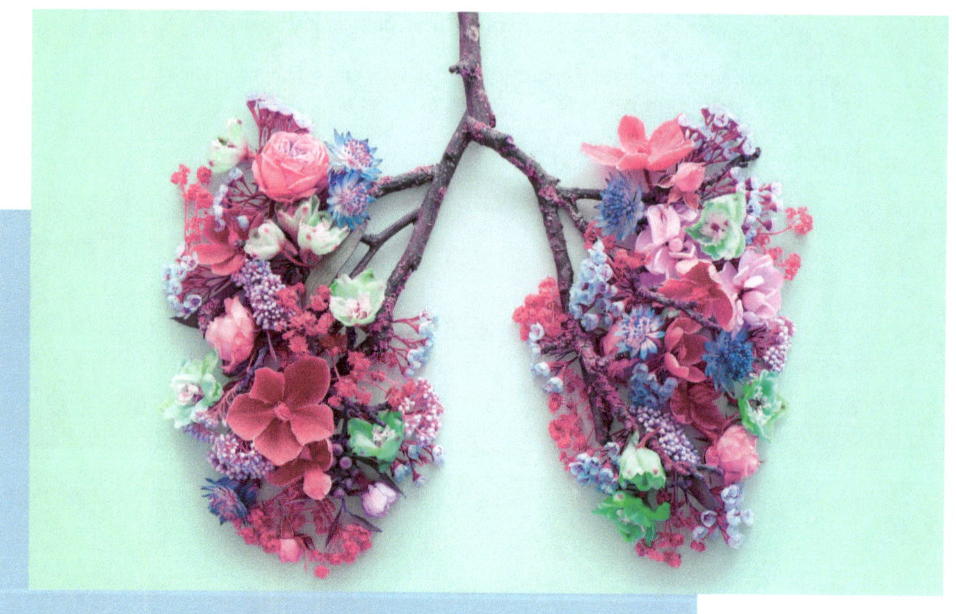

BREATHING

Amazing fact: Even if you are legitimately stressed out because situations in your life are overwhelming, you can trick your brain into believing that you are okay, just by breathing.

Let's talk about how and why.

We all know that in times of stress, we are programmed for fight, flight or freeze responses. When these responses begin, we either stop breathing, (freeze) or start to breathe very quicky (fight or flight). Evolutionary Scientists (no- not just the we-came-from-monkeys ones, but also the our-bodies-develop-mechanisms-to-help-us-survive ones) say it makes total sense. If we are being hunted, and need to freeze to stay hidden, we will also stop breathing, to be as quiet as possible. If we need to flee from danger or fight a predator, our breathing accelerates, oxygenating our body as our heart pumps blood through our system at full speed. We are primed and ready to go.

If there was danger, our breathing would be accelerated, or stopped. Our bodies know this. So. when we consciously slow our breathing, keep it steady and strong, our brain understands that there must be no danger and our stress hormones (cortisol levels) go down, And then- we feel better. It is so simple.

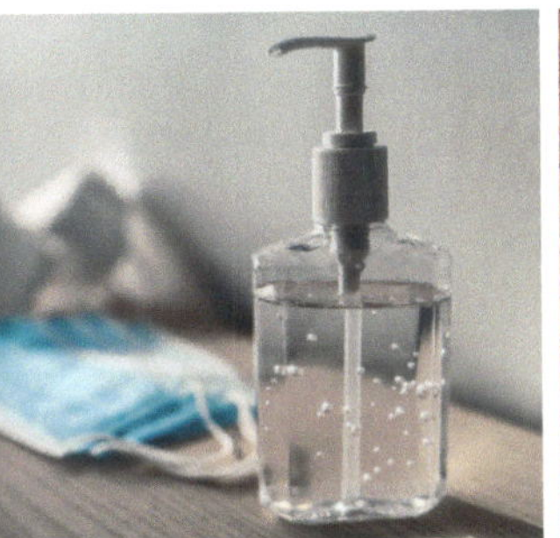
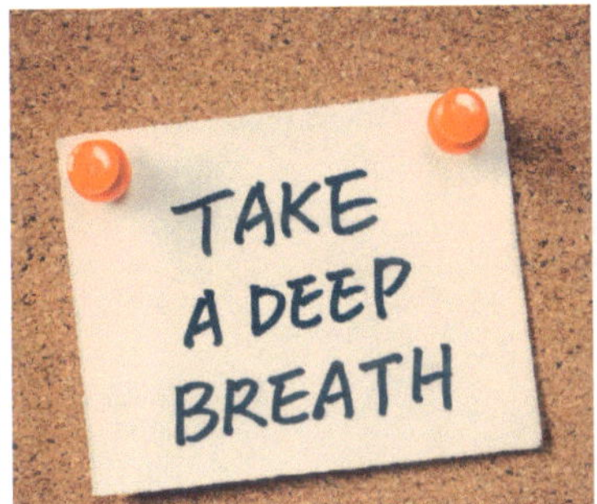

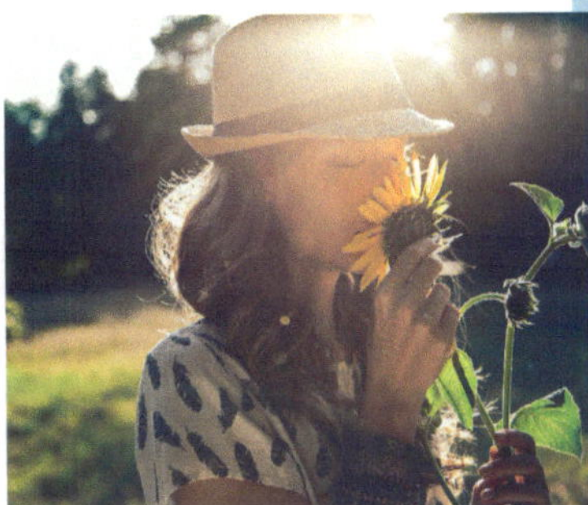

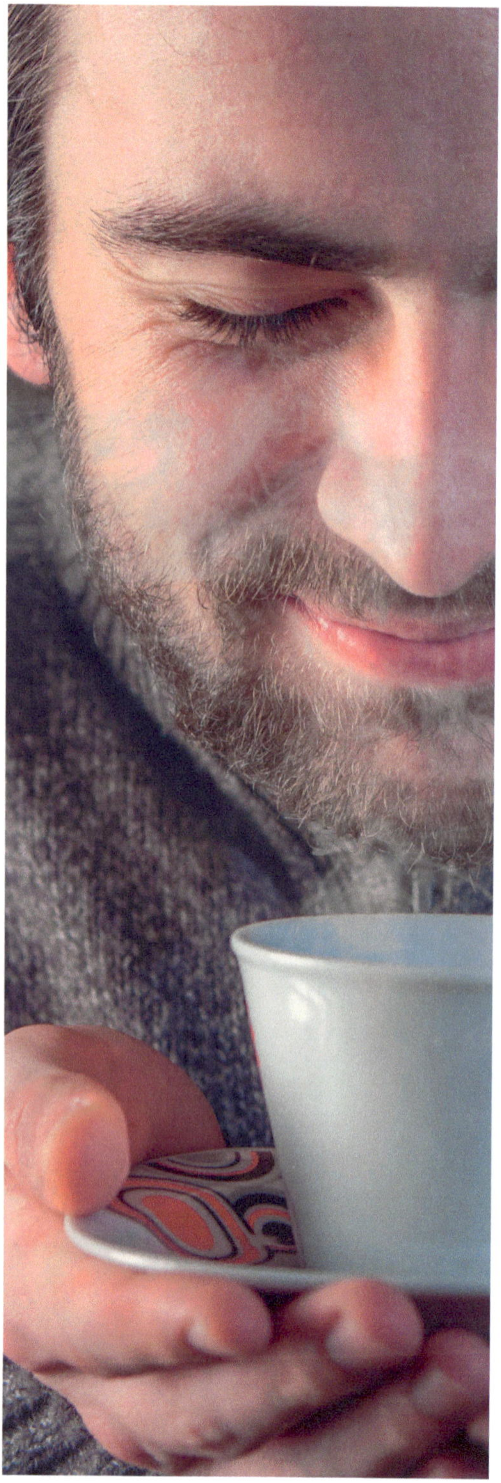

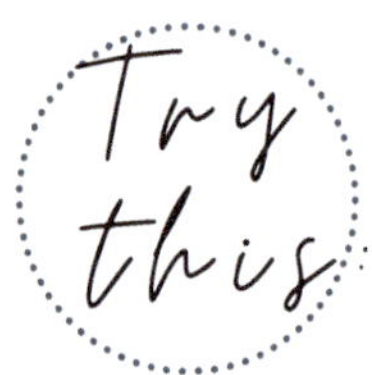

I read a children's book a while ago with some great breathing exercises.

My favorite goes as follows. Read it all, and then take a moment to try. Notice your body and how you feel, before and after the exercise.

I want you to close your eyes, and just breathe for a moment. Breathe in, nice and deep, and then breathe out. I want you to feel your feet, how they touch the floor, and your back, against the chair. Listen to the sounds around you. Keep breathing.

Now in your minds eye, I want you to imagine that you are holding a cup of hot chocolate. The mug warms your hands, the temperature is just right.

You lean over the cup and inhale deeply, imagine how that chocolate smells, breathe it in and savor it.

Now blow gently, lips pursed, as if you are cooling the drink before sipping. A nice, long, cooling breath out, through your mouth.

Repeat this for a couple of minutes. Breathing in through your nose, aroma filling your lungs and imagination, and then out through your mouth, blowing the steam from the cup, creating little ripples as you exhale.

The wonderful thing about this exercise is that we already know exactly how to do this. Breathe in, breathe out. Try it now.

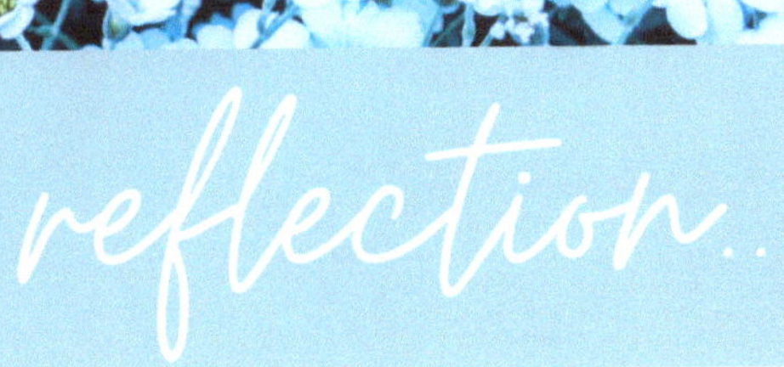

What I tried: ____

How I felt before the exercise: _______________________________

____

____

How I felt afterward: _______________________________________

____

____

What I liked about it: ______________________________________

____

____

What I didn't like about it: _________________________________

____

____

Additional thoughts: _______________________________________

____

Would I try it again? ____________________________________

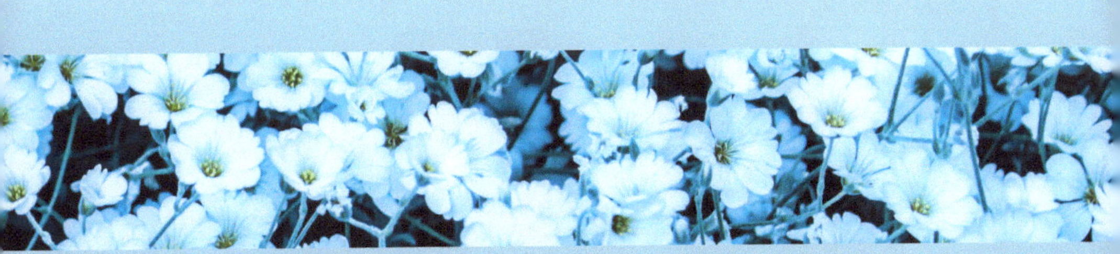

Notes

TWO: GROUND

2

"If you must look back, do so forgivingly. If you must look forward, do so prayerfully. However, the wisest thing you can do is to be present in the present. Gratefully."

-Maya Angelou

Grounding is a word that has many meanings. Being "grounded" can mean your parents won't let you leave your room or it can mean placing your feet literally on the earth to allow its electrical forces to positively affect your body. Grounding can also describe a safety precaution when dealing with electricity. The grounding I'm talking about is the act of intentionally focusing on the present moment, usually by using your senses, which is an effective calming exercise when you are experiencing negative or challenging emotions.

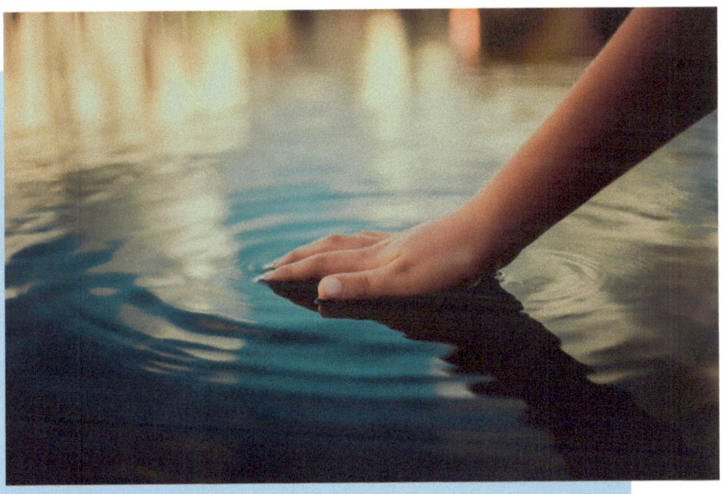

GROUNDING

I don't know about you, but sometimes I have a hard time staying in the moment. It is so easy for me to get sucked into painful memories or regret from my past, or to just worry, worry, worry about the future.

Even if- in this moment- everything is okay, I can spend hours regretting that I didn't parent my kids better as they grew up, or worrying that I won't have financial security in my old age.

What I'm doing in those moments is trading the peace of the present for the burden of the past and the uncertainty of the future. What a terrible trade.

When we practice grounding, we use our five senses and tangible objects to anchor us in the present- the here and now- to help us move through difficult moments.

Grounding can effectively help us to escape panic attacks, the urge to self-harm, unwanted memories, anxiety, and more.

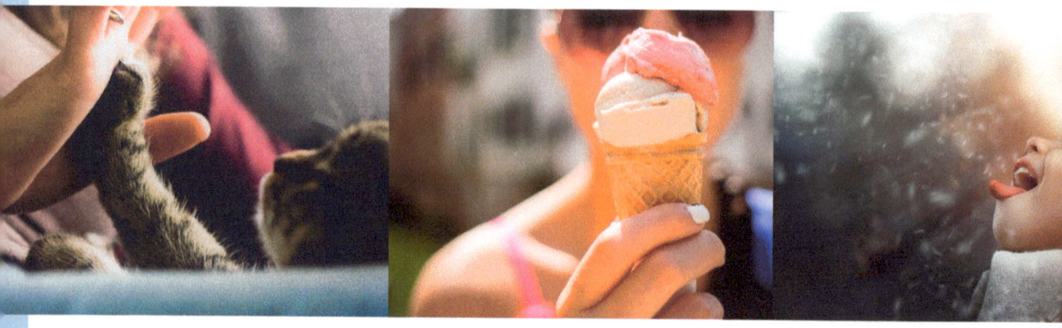

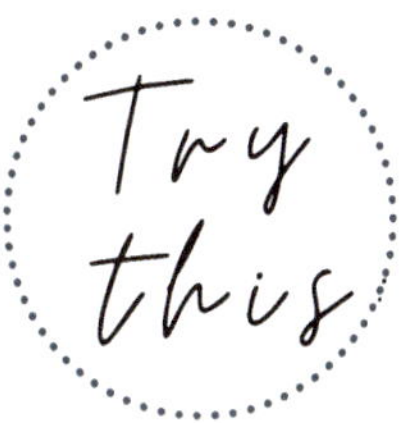

There are so many grounding techniques, if these ones don't work well for you, don't give up finding one that does. None of them are difficult, and they really can feel like a life-saver when you are feeling swept away by emotion- no matter where you are. Here are two of my favorites.

5,4,3,2,1

For this exercise, you are going to engage all of your senses. Wherever you are, in school, in the mall, driving, I want you to list (out loud or in your head) -

5 things you can see. (Sale signs, smile of a friend, your hands, the stars, etc.)

4 things you can feel. (Your gloves on your fingers, heartbeat, grunge on your teeth, itchy tag, etc.)

3 things you can hear. (The furnace running, tap dripping, footsteps of passerby, your own breathing, etc.)

2 things you can smell. (Popcorn, fresh air, grass, even body odor)

and **1** thing you can taste. That's it. You will find your focus shifts.

Find the color

This is so easy, and has helped 100% of the friends who have tried it. All you do is **choose a color-** let's say orange- and name (in your head or out loud) everything you can see that is orange. "I see an orange sign, I see an orange stripe on that car. I see orange pants... " Notice how quickly you return to the present, and how your body relaxes.

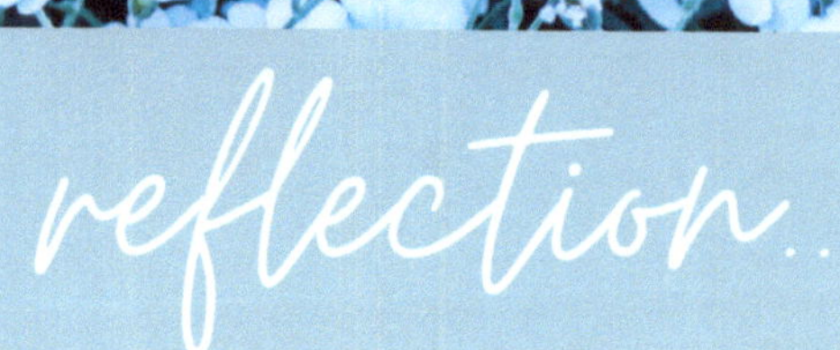

reflection...

What I tried: _______________________________

How I felt before the exercise: _______________________________

____

____

How I felt afterward: _______________________________

____

____

What I liked about it: _______________________________

____

____

What I didn't like about it: _______________________________

____

____

Additional thoughts: _______________________________

____

Would I try it again? _______________________________

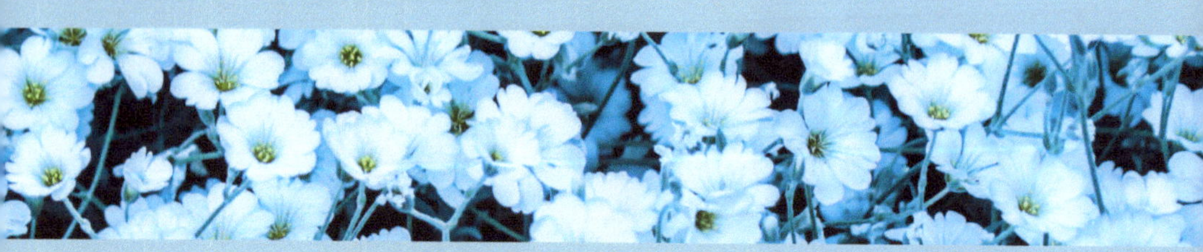

Notes

THREE: GET AWAY

"We need quiet time to examine our lives openly and honestly – spending quiet time alone gives your mind an opportunity to renew itself and create order."
– Susan L. Taylor

How often do you hear someone say "I just need to get away from it all!" How often do *you* feel that way?

Sometimes life is exhausting, especially since Covid changed our world. Suddenly we had to adapt to both home learning and doing our work from home, If you're a parent, you had a lot of time with your kids, adjusting to each other's full time presence. Our homes are full of duties and obligations. There is always something to be done, or someone to be helped, and when we finally sit down, the news or social media can suck the rest of our energy right out of us. We really do need to get away.

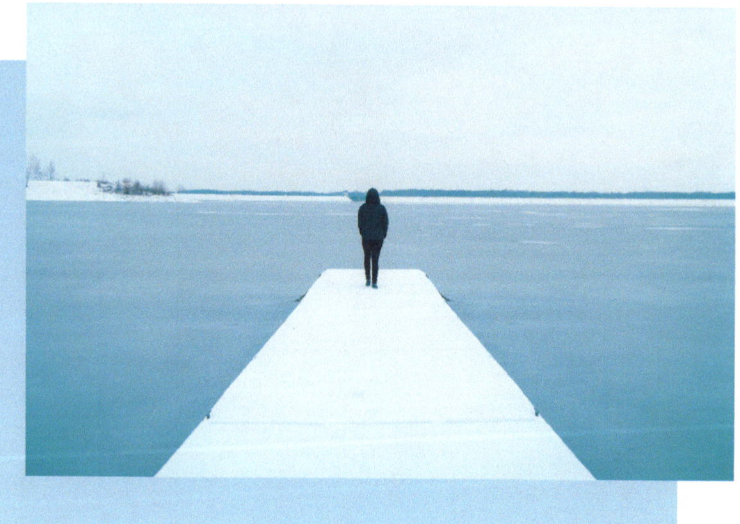

GET AWAY

There have been a few times in my life where I just wasn't functioning. I felt like I was trying to do it all- but I was doing it all very poorly. Parenting, schooling, friendships, creative endeavors, finances, housework... it was all too much. I needed to get away.

Getting away can look different for everyone, and it's important to "get away" in a way that allows your mind to rest. Literal space from your work or worries is important to regain some perspective. When we're too close to stress, stress is all we can see.

When my kids were little, my version of getting away was having a bath. If my mood was low or I wasn't coping well, I would sometimes run three or four baths a day. I would sit in the aromatic water, let the heat blanket me, and just be alone. My children would sometimes knock at the door, or lay on the floor outside the bathroom, tiny voices bouncing over the linoleum, They learned that this was mom time, and they could talk to me in 20 minutes, or go find their dad.

As my kids became teenagers (and one of them inherited my bathing habit), I needed a new way to get away. This time I called it my mental health walk. My job was to put on shoes and go out the door. That was it. If I came home in three minutes, no guilt. Most of the time I walked for an hour or so. I breathed fresh air, I watched the leaves dance across the street, and listened to the magpies croak to one another. I always felt better after that little getaway.

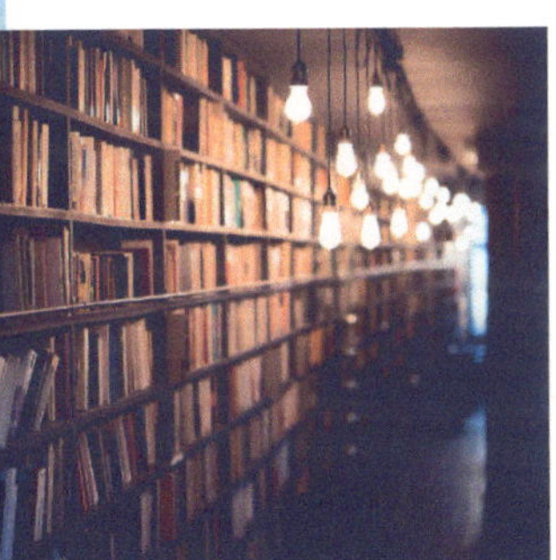
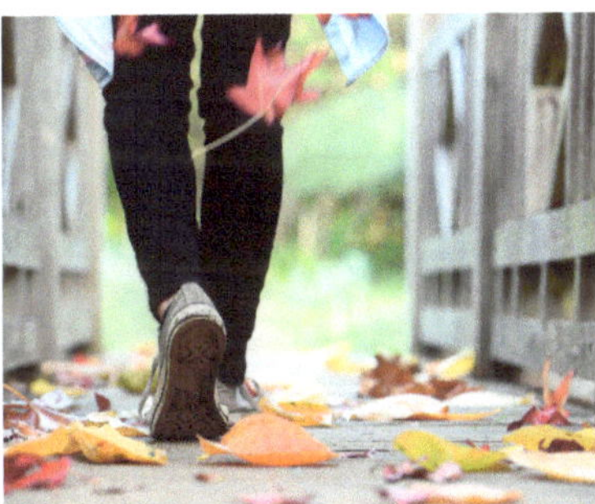
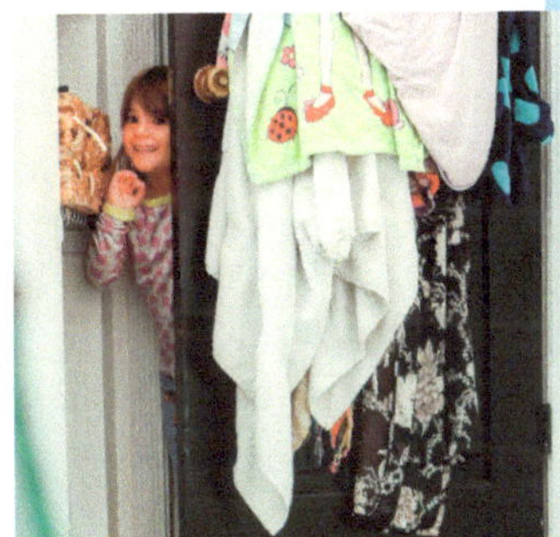

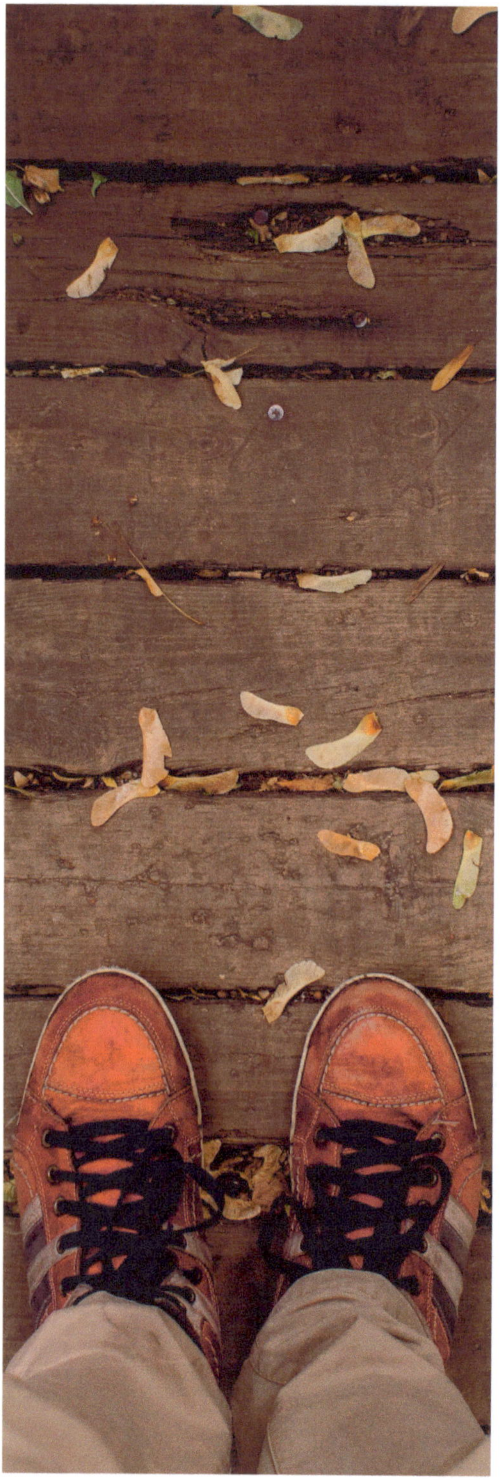

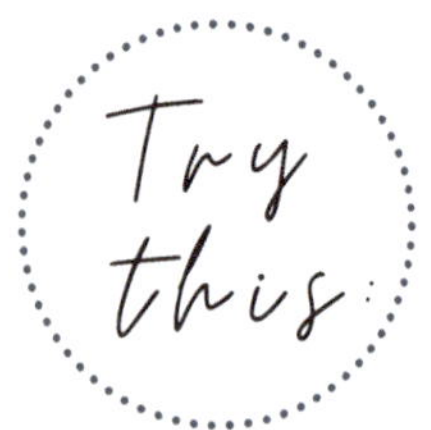

How you "get away" is personal.

Take a moment and think about what you need.

Do you need quiet?

Do you need action?

Do you need physical activity?

If you're not sure, try some of these suggestions, and see what works. Use your getaway time to relax your mind. Do your best to stay in the moment, and leave home at home.

Put on those shoes and try the mental health walk. Just go.

Close the door to your room and pick up that book you bought ages ago and never read.

Head to your front or back steps, maybe a deck if you have one, and watch the sky for a while.

Hop in the car and drive somewhere that's interesting to you. Park and observe the world as it moves.

Hit the mall, and if you can, treat yourself to your favorite drink. Enjoy it as you let your mind wander.

Walk in nature.

Go for a massage.

For any of these activities, try not to feel rushed. Set aside time, and then take it.

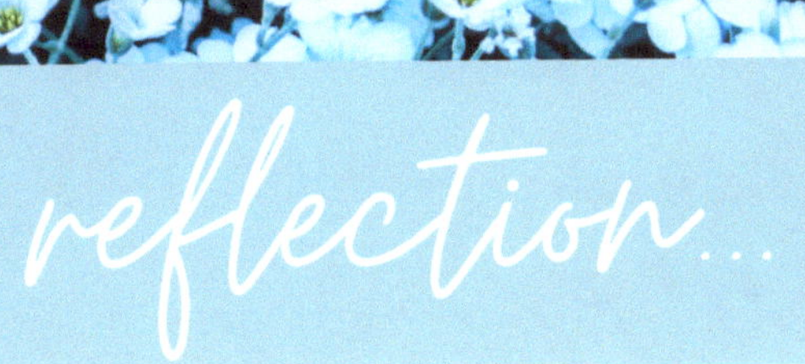

What I tried: _______________________________________

How I felt before the exercise: _______________________
____
____

How I felt afterward: _________________________________
____
____

What I liked about it: ________________________________
____
____

What I didn't like about it: ___________________________
____
____

Additional thoughts: _________________________________
____

Would I try it again? ______________________________

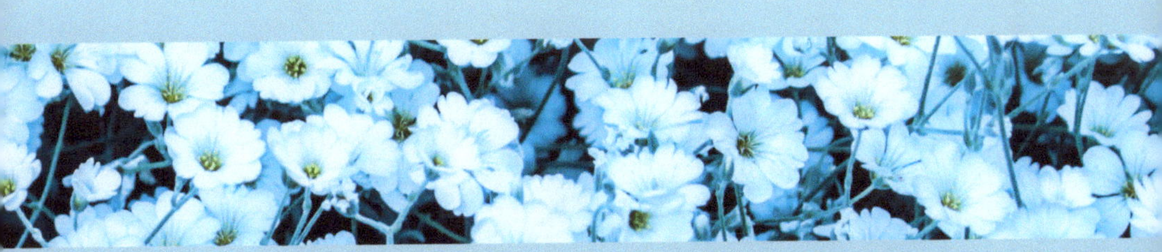

Notes

FOUR: REST

4

"If you get tired, learn to rest, not to quit."
-Bansk

Maybe getting away feels like a rest. But getting away and resting are not necessarily the same thing. Both of these steps involve creating time for yourself, which is difficult in the ever-demanding world we live in.

Even if you can't get away, you must find a way to rest.

So what is rest?

According to the Oxford dictionary, **rest** is to : **cease work or movement in order to relax, refresh oneself, or recover strength.** "He needed to rest after the feverish activity." OR to: **be placed or supported so as to stay in a specified position.** "Her elbow was resting on the arm of the sofa."

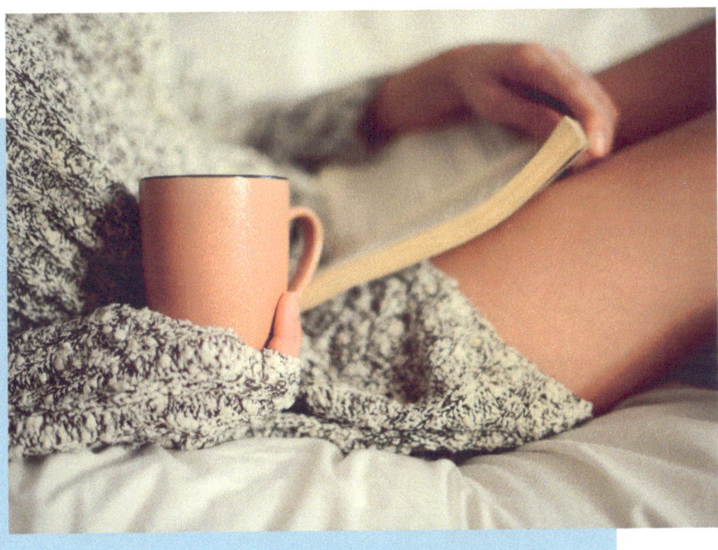

REST

I really like the second definition. It's not really the kind of rest I'm describing, but the idea of being supported in order to hold your position seems incredibly relevant.

Recently I heard a wise Tiktok-er tell me that rest is not a reward. This statement stopped me in my tracks. Why? Because I totally treat rest like a reward. If I get such and such done, then I can sit down for a bit with a coffee. Sometimes it sounds like... "When I finish the dishes, and getting the kids to bed, and I've packed their lunches for tomorrow, and switched the laundry, and", and, and. The list just keeps getting longer. If we try to earn rest, we'll never actually find it. Instead, we have to make rest a priority so we are better able to accomplish the things we have to do, sanity intact.

We only have so many hours in a day, and 'making time' seems like a silly phrase. We cannot actually make time. But. We can reserve time for rest, just like we do for so many other important things.

Sometimes we have to take some good things off of our list, in order to do the best ones. We cannot do it all. And when we try, we end up hating ourselves because we're not doing any of it as well as we want to. We also forget that the world will continue to revolve without us. Someone else will drive the kids, make the signs, or cook dinner. But not until we give it up.

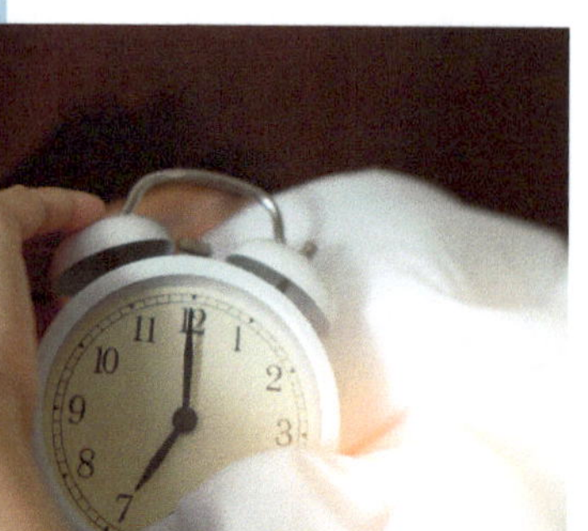
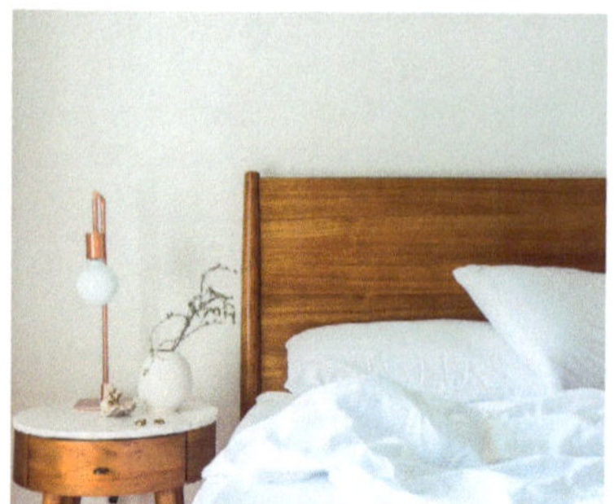
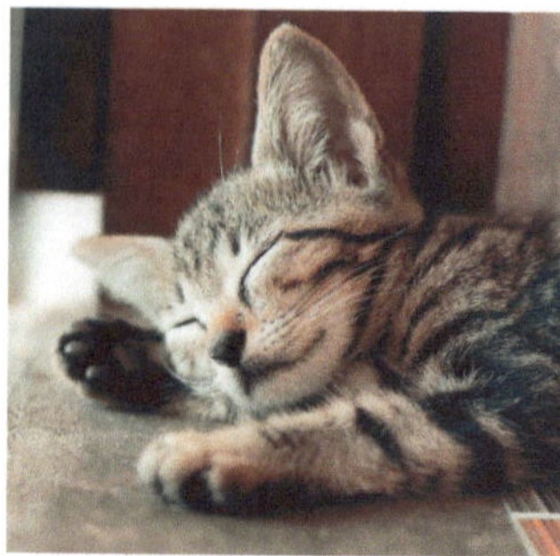

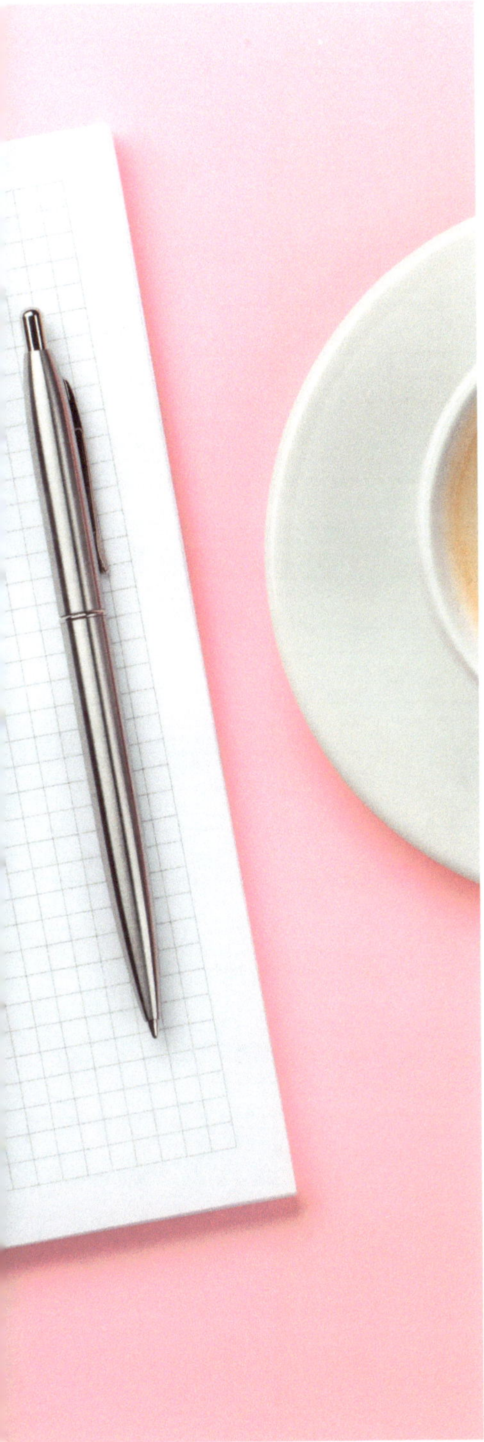

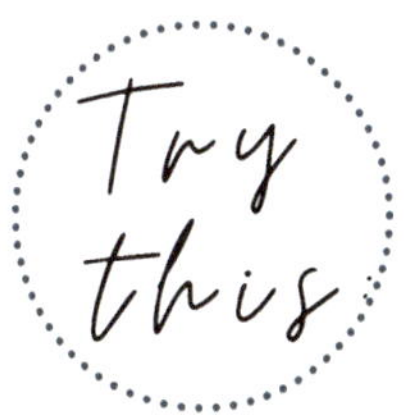

If you are a list maker, this will come naturally. If not, try it anyway.

I want you to make a list of all the things you would usually do in your day. You may feel like you'll be writing forever, but try to include things that wouldn't usually make it onto an official to-do list. Things like making dinner, cleaning up after dinner, shoveling the snow, driving the kids to school, calling a friend, even having a shower.

When you're done, have a look at it and give yourself a pat on the back. You are a freaking superhero. Look at all those things.

I understand that you may not get them all done every day, but that is a whole lot of things on your shoulders.

Now look at that list and see if any of those things could be called 'rest'.

If yes, (maybe a bath, or nap) good for you. I wonder if those are the things that get pushed down the list as the day runs short.

Now look at your list and try to identify 2 things that you could designate to someone else, or that you don't need to do everyday. What could you put in its place that might give you a moment of rest?

The next list you make- put something restful on it. Lay on the couch and listen to music, do some gentle stretching, hold your pet.

Make it a priority, and see what changes.

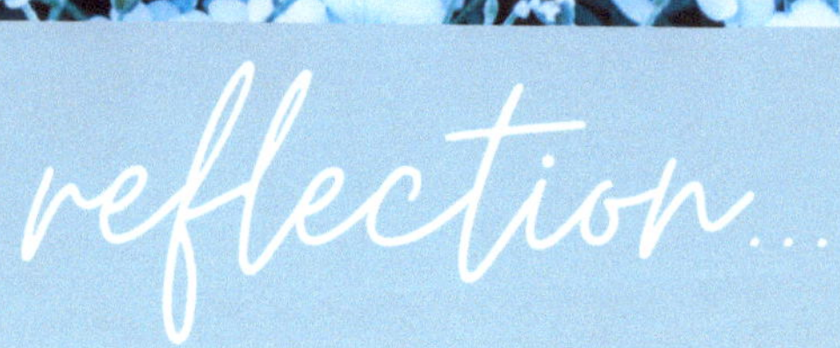

reflection...

What I tried: ___________________________________

How I felt before the exercise: ___________________
____
____

How I felt afterward: ______________________________
____
____

What I liked about it: ______________________________
____
____

What I didn't like about it: ________________________
____
____

Additional thoughts: _______________________________
____

Would I try it again? ___________________________

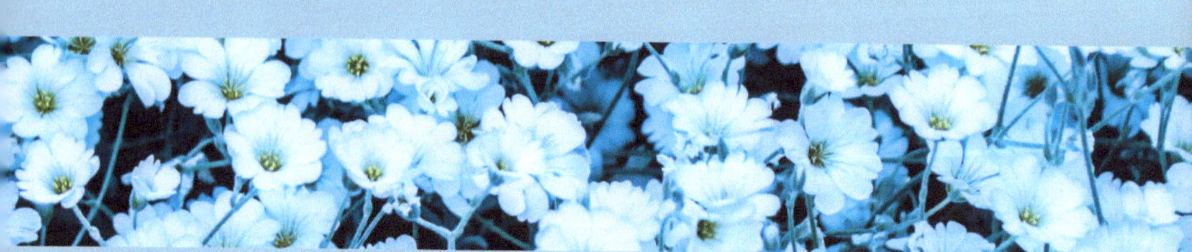

Notes

FIVE: NOTICE YOUR IMPACT

"Every action we take impacts the lives of others around us."
-Arthur Carmazzi

Hopefully you've found some time to get away, and to rest. If you have, your brain will be wandering. You may struggle to keep it from worry and stress.

Use this moment to think about your place in this world. Think about how your actions change the lives of the people around you. Friends, family, neighbours, coworkers, even strangers in passing. Make no mistake, your life affects others.

Sometimes our actions or reactions are the start of a ripple effect. It may start as something small or it might start with a splash, but those rippling rings reach well beyond the initial point of impact.

Are the ripples positive? What kind of difference are you making?

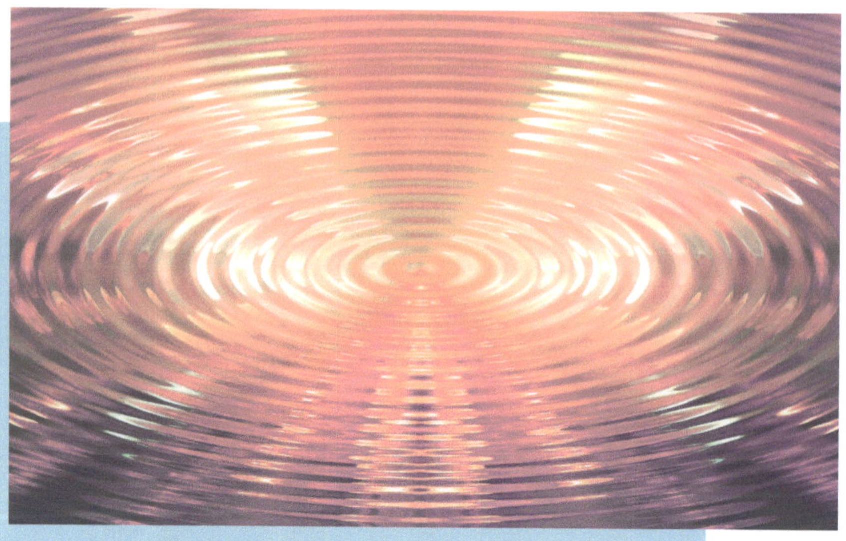

NOTICE YOUR IMPACT

Most of us have experienced the pay it forward phenomenon. Something great happens to you, or is given to you, and the giver simply wants you to be kind to someone else, when and however you can. It's a great ripple movement, a beautiful thing to see and to be a part of. We all know, however, that that our impact can happen in other ways, too.

When we're not okay, it usually shows, and it affects the people around us. You might be sprinkling your sadness, anger, detachment or fear as you go about your everyday life- without even knowing it. It is so important to be aware of how we affect the world.

Instead of feeling guilty for any negative vibes you might be sharing, congratulate yourself on noticing your impact, and ask yourself- what could you do to bring more peace, joy, or positivity to those same people in your life?

Perhaps all you do is pour out. The only thing you think about it whether that ripple is big enough or effective enough. You try and try and are exhausted. Breathe, my friend. You are not the only one out there that is contributing. You may need to make sure that the farther reaching ripples are not in fact taking much needed love and attention from the ones nearer to you. Your home, family, your best friends; they may be losing out. Check in and see.

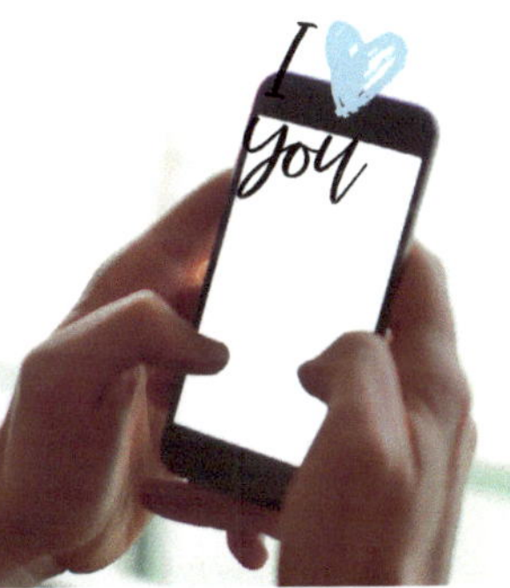

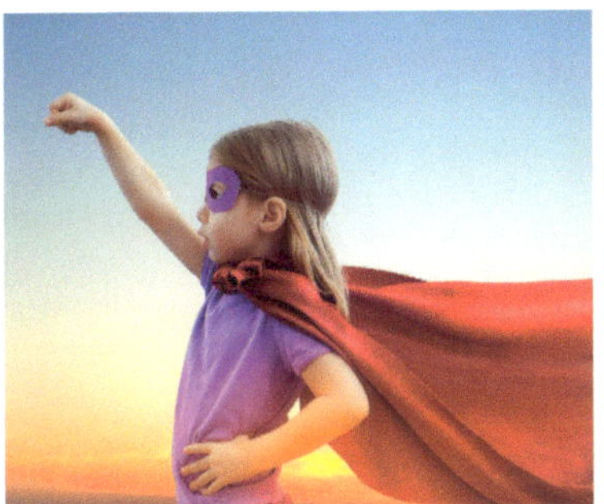

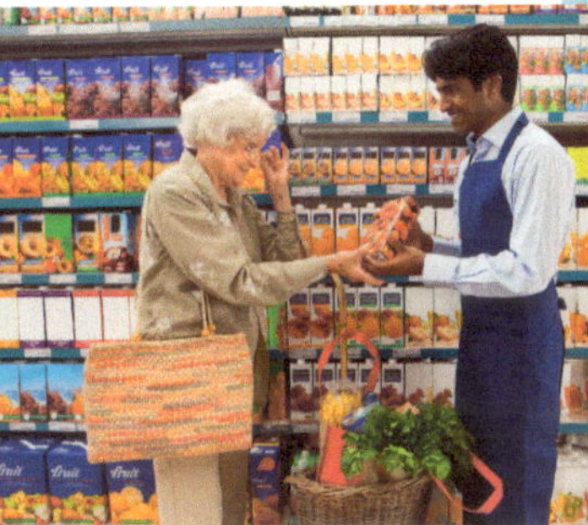

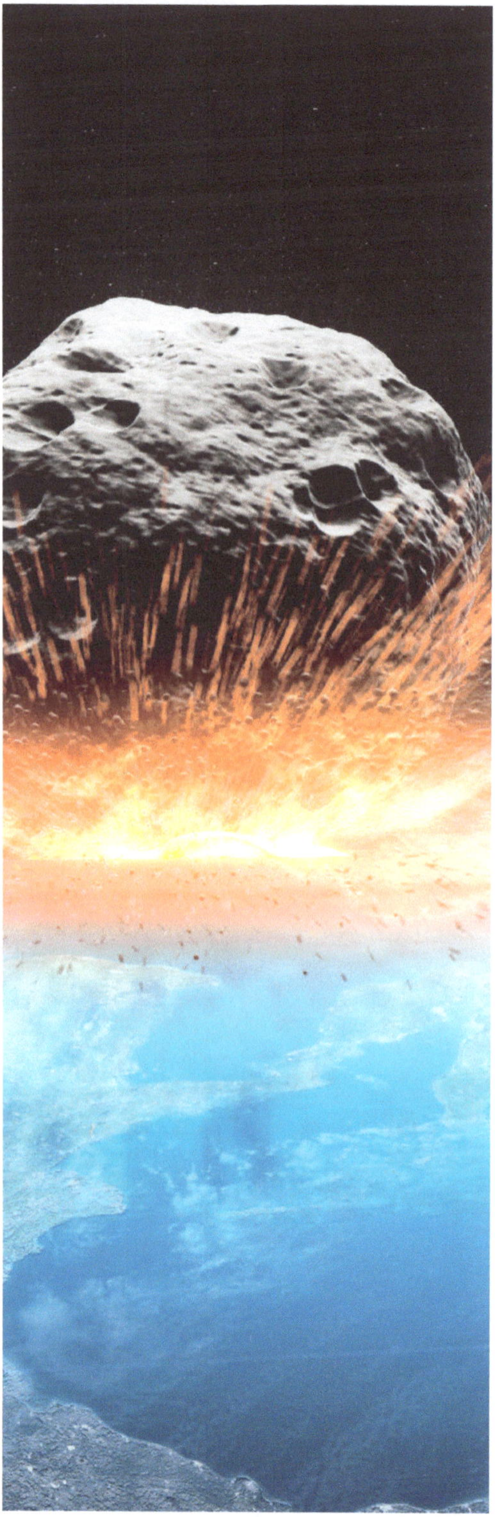

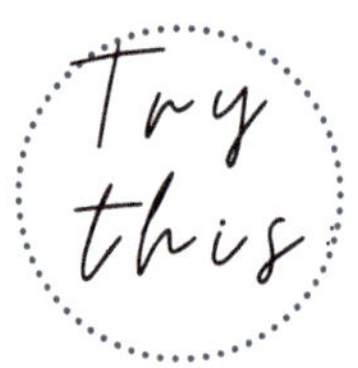

Most of the time our impact on others goes largely unnoticed by our own selves. We gesture angrily to another (inconsiderate) driver and go on with our day. We reach a box of Kleenex from the top shelf at the grocery store for a gentleman in a wheelchair. We nod mutely as our child chatters about the video game they just conquered while scrolling on our phone or returning a text, and we kiss our beloved on the forehead before bed. Each interaction creates a reaction that is absorbed, carried, and most often passed on to someone else. Do we understand the power we have in those moments?

Take a few moments and think about some of the interactions that have affected your life. Did a friend call in a lonely moment? Did a stranger compliment your outfit as you walked into a job interview? Maybe you bought something online and found out you were cheated, or struggled to stand on the bus with your groceries, while others sat and ignored you. Some of the smallest things can have the greatest impact, good or bad.

Now think about you. How do you treat people? Are you present enough in the moment to notice? What is the ripple effect that is widening around you on a daily basis?

If you can, spend the evening 'watching' your own self. Try to be with family, or friends, or even out in a public place. Notice your actions and reactions, and watch for the response of others around you.

Then do something or say something intentionally kind, and see what happens.

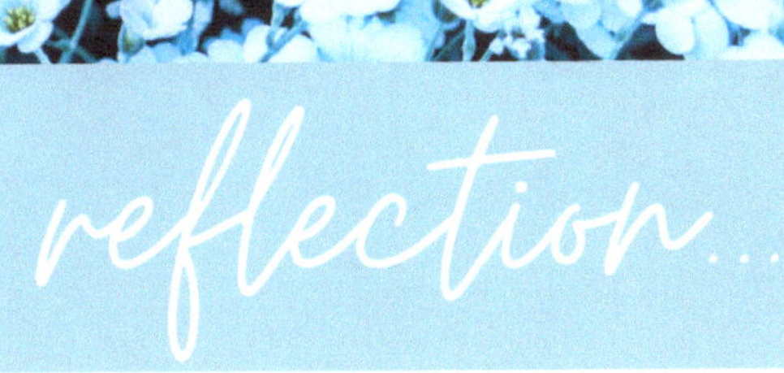

What I tried: ____

How I felt before the exercise: _________________________________

____

____

How I felt afterward: ____

____

____

What I liked about it: ____

____

____

What I didn't like about it: ____________________________________

____

____

Additional thoughts: ____

____

Would I try it again? ____

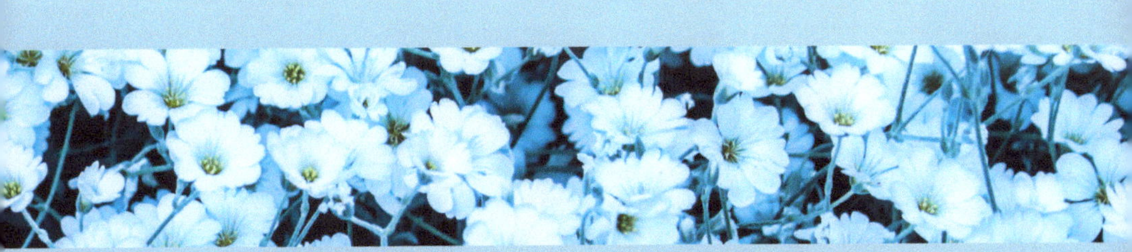

Notes

SIX: CREATE

6

"In a time of destruction, create something."
— Maxine Hong Kingston

We are creative beings. Even the most linear of human thinkers, will create in his or her own way. I remember watching my dad draw a beautiful lion and hearing him insist that he was not an artist. His rationale? Because his technique wasn't "flowy". He created with a mathematical precision, seeing an animal broken into replicable parts, and then he replicated them.

Creation is in us. And when life gets heavy, creating fills our troubles with helium, lifts them from your backs, and allows us to forget about them for a while.

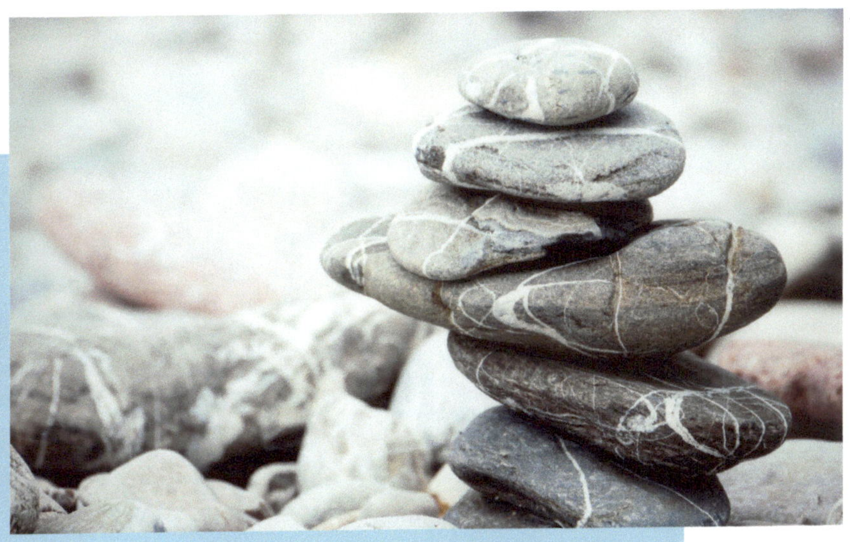

CREATE

When we hear the word create, most of us think art. We think of crafts, and writing, and painting, and for sure those things are creative outlets for many of us. Some write songs, some dance, some weave.

But creating is so much more than that. Creating is bringing something into existence that wasn't here before.

I had a friend once that never used recipes. She would throw in seemingly random ingredients, cook them up, and feed everyone. It always tasted good. I remember one day she called me. She said "Char! You would be so proud of me! I made muffins and I even followed the recipe!" I laughed as she continued. "Except I used applesauce instead of sugar, and I put in some yogurt too!" You know what? They were wonderful. She created with ingredients. Flavour, combination, presentation. It brought her life.

My daughters enjoy makeup, and building beautiful looks just for fun. My son loves to take pictures of everyday things, but from an unusual perspective. Some people love math equations, some stacking stones, some Lego building, some computer coding, websites or creating programs or activities to help people. There are limitless options.

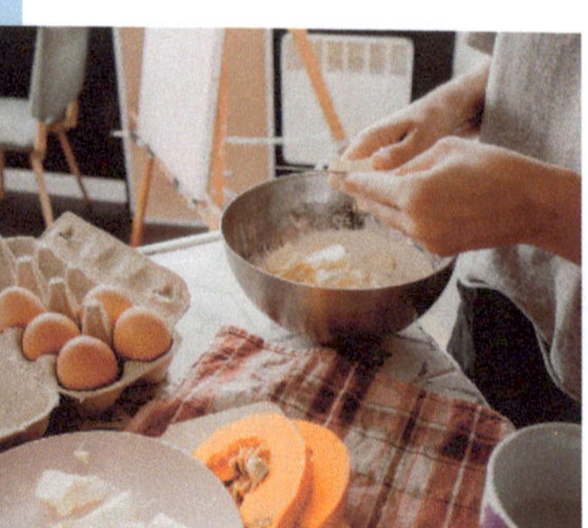
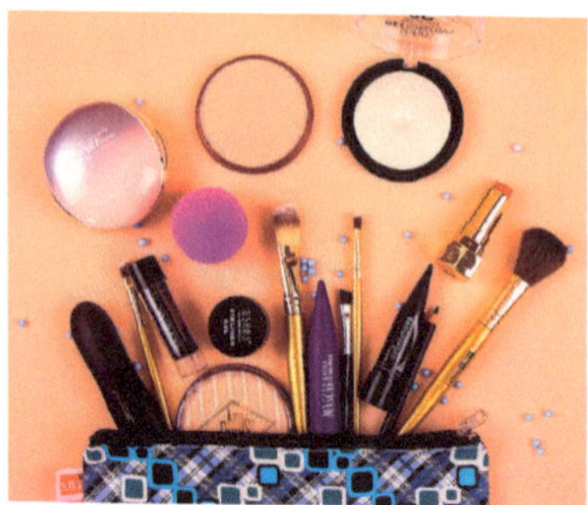
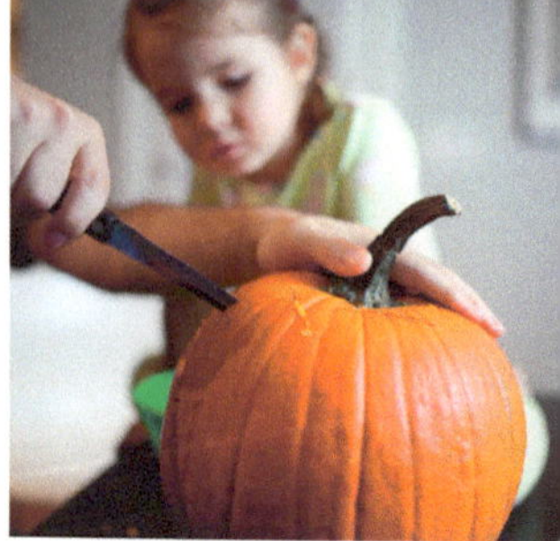

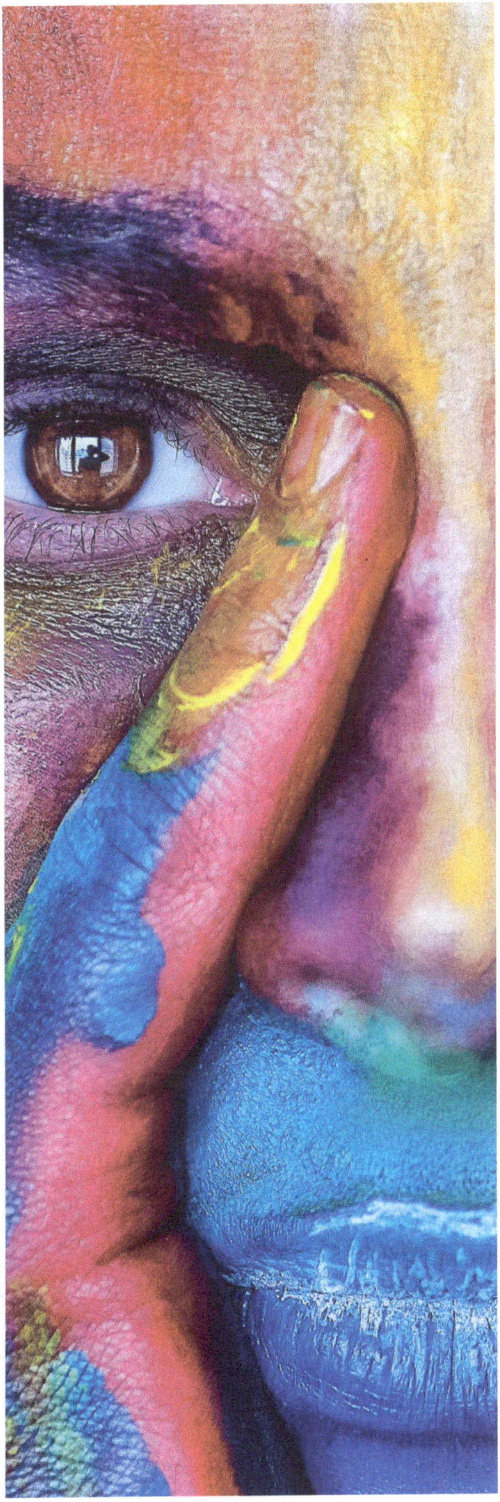

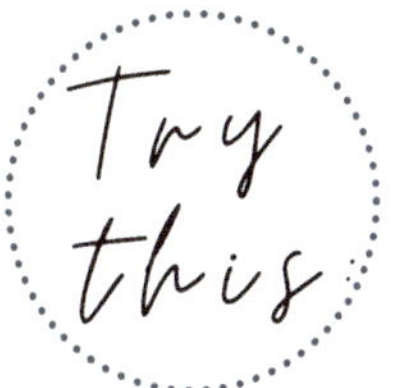

Ready? GO!

Think of something that you've always wanted to try or something that you love doing but never make time for (yes I said never *make* time, not never *have* time) and do it.

Remember to keep it achievable. Don't decide to paint a portrait if you have no paint or paper (unless you want to get even more creative). Don't aim to complete an afghan if you've never crocheted a dishcloth. Start small, and work your way up. It's the process that counts.

Breathe and smile. Breathe and smile. Breathe and smile.

Rules for creating:

1 Be kind to yourself. Our focus for creating is the process, not the finished product. Oftentimes we end up with something totally different than we were planning, but it is still valuable. Reserve judgement.

2. Try, Try again. (don't give up)

3. Two are better than one. Ask someone to join you.

4. There are no rules. Haha. Other than these ones, of course. When you are creating, you can rethink things, repeat things or do things differently. It doesn't matter how anyone else does it, you are creating! Do it your way, and enjoy learning.

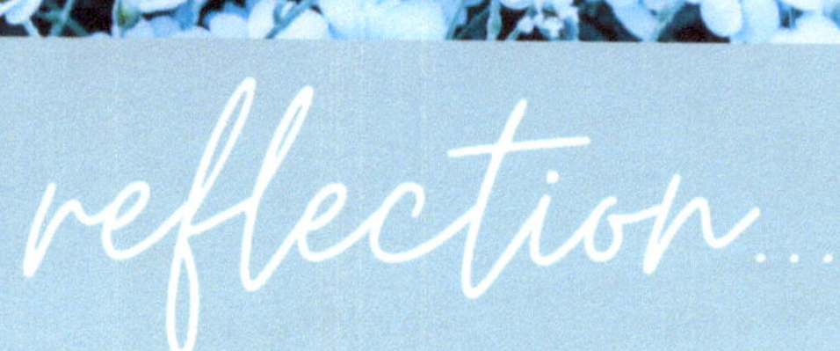

reflection...

What I tried: _______________________

How I felt before the exercise: _______________________
____
____

How I felt afterward: _______________________
____
____

What I liked about it: _______________________
____
____

What I didn't like about it: _______________________
____
____

Additional thoughts: _______________________
____

Would I try it again? _______________________

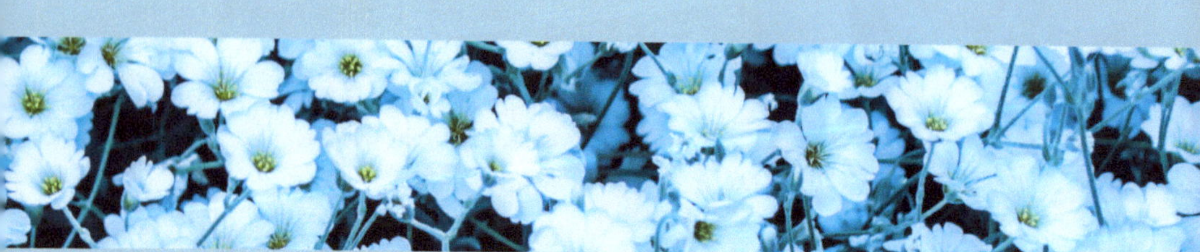

Notes

SEVEN: CONNECT

7

"We are like islands in the sea, separate on the surface but connected in the deep."
-William James

In a world that offers more ways to connect than ever before, we are somehow a society that is also more lonely than ever before. Sure, we may feel connected to that tiktok personality that speaks to us like they know us, and brings daily laughs or encouragement, but the reality is- they don't know us, and in a moment of loneliness, we can't call them up or ask them for a hug. We may have 500 Facebook "friends", but do they notice if you stop posting for a few days? Do they know anything about you that you haven't posted for the world to see? And c'mon, we all know that we carefully curate the things that we post, good, bad, and ugly. There are many, many things we don't share with the wide world.

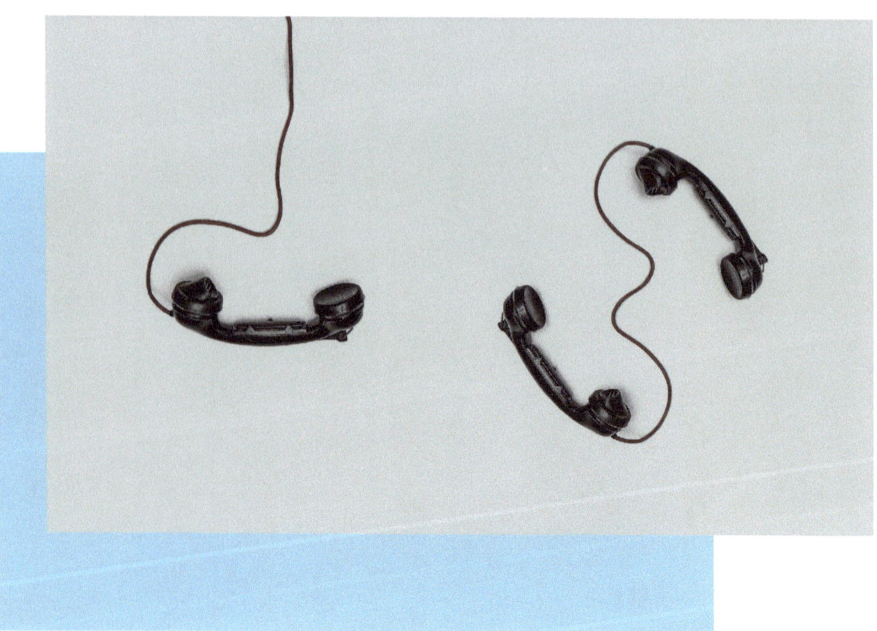

CONNECT

Humans were born to connect, physically and emotionally. Studies show that babies without human connection do not thrive, and that proves true throughout our lifetime. There is a deep need within each of us to belong, to be seen and heard, and to be touched. As we experience life, our needs can grow and change, but in some way we will always need that connection in order to thrive.

Years ago, I had separated from my then-husband and was not in a relationship. I had four kids, 3/4 were teenagers who did not want hugs or cuddles from me although they enjoyed spending time with me. I remember one particular day, I was in the car with my sister-in-law, and I was expressing how much I missed human touch after almost a year of being alone. Intentionally, with great love, she held out her hand to me. I took it and we held hands while we drove around our little town. I cried. I felt loved. She had met my need for physical connection.

For me it was touch, but for some it's being heard. Someone that listens and understands, validates your experience. Sometimes it might be re-connecting with someone from your past who has always meant a lot to you, and whom you haven't spent much time with. Those people that always bring you rest and make you smile. You connect. You feel better.

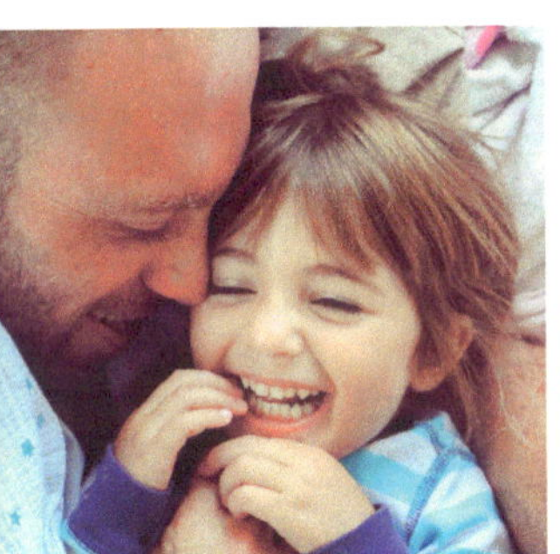
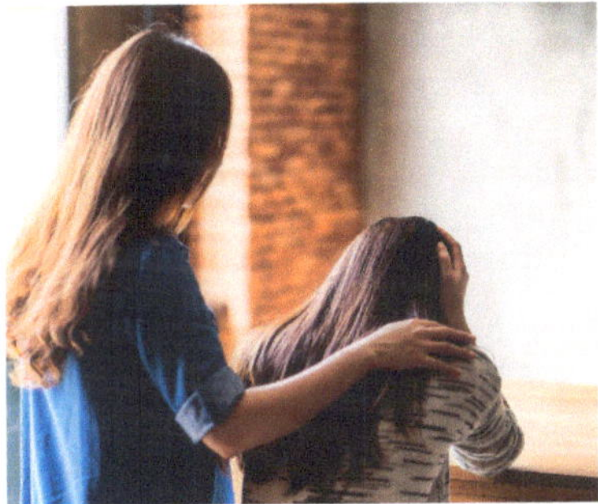
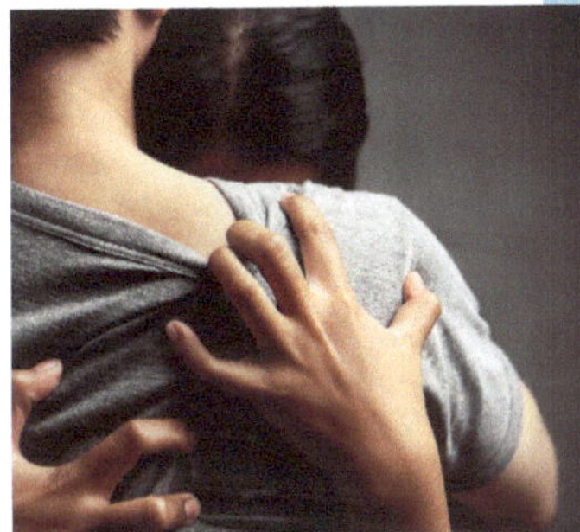

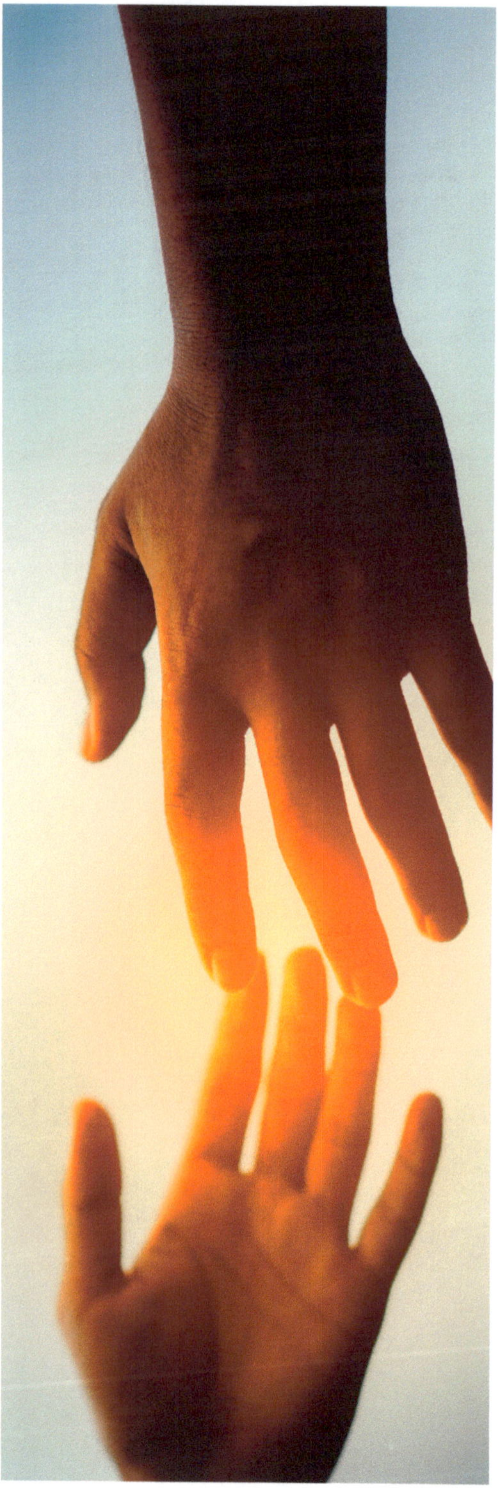

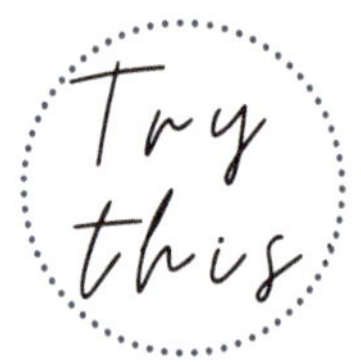

Take a moment to think about what kind of connections you have, and what kinds you might need. Then choose a way to meet one of those needs. Try it out and see how it works for you. If the need remains unmet, try something different.

Here are a few ideas of how to meet connection needs:

Physical:
Hold a pet, close to your chest if possible.
Hold the hand of a safe person.
Ask for a hug from someone that you know is a hugger. Be held for as long as they'll hold you, or as long as you're comfortable.

If actual physical contact with other people isn't possible, close your eyes and imagine it. Imagine your hand in theirs, or your head resting on their chest. Or put your hand on your own heart. You will still experience some of the benefits of connection.

Emotional:
Call or get together with a friend or family member- one that you know is a good listener, and will validate your feelings.
Call a crisis or help line, or join a support group. Sometimes we don't have a friend that can understand, but there is someone out there that does. Find them. Talk to someone that relates and allows you to connect through shared experiences.

Spiritual:
Listen to music that connects you.
Pray.
Go to a place of worship.
Go outside.

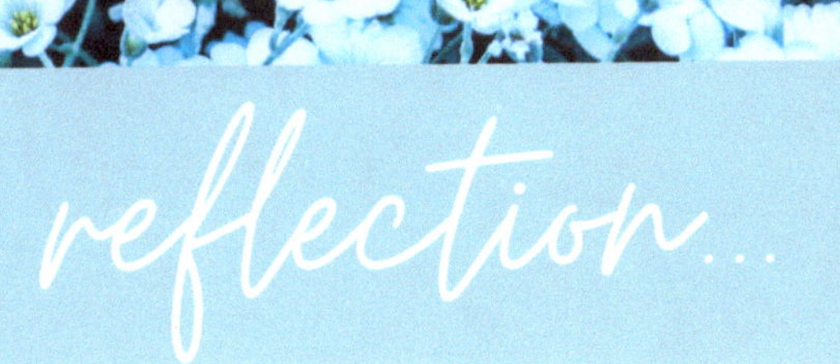

What I tried: ____

How I felt before the exercise: _________________________________

____

____

How I felt afterward: ____

____

____

What I liked about it: ____

____

____

What I didn't like about it: ____________________________________

____

____

Additional thoughts: ____

____

Would I try it again? ____

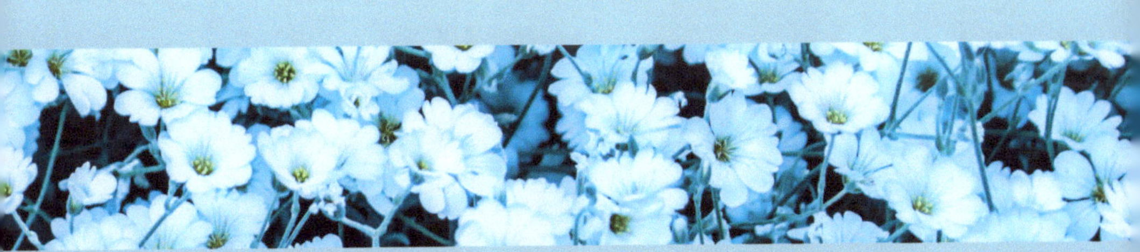

Notes

EIGHT: PRAY/GIVE IT UP

"Give it to God, and go to sleep."
-Unknown

Trigger Warning re: suicide.

I have had many, many nights where my one of my children were struggling. Sometimes with some really big things. Things that I couldn't solve, couldn't resolve. Painful, scary, scarring things.

Sometimes they were so overwhelmed they wanted to die.

I have four beautiful kids, and was parenting on my own. I also worked full time. I could not stay up every night to make sure my children stayed alive. I know that probably sounds awful, but it's true. I never went to bed when they were in high crisis, but I did go to bed, and the terror of waking up and finding them dead was very, very real.

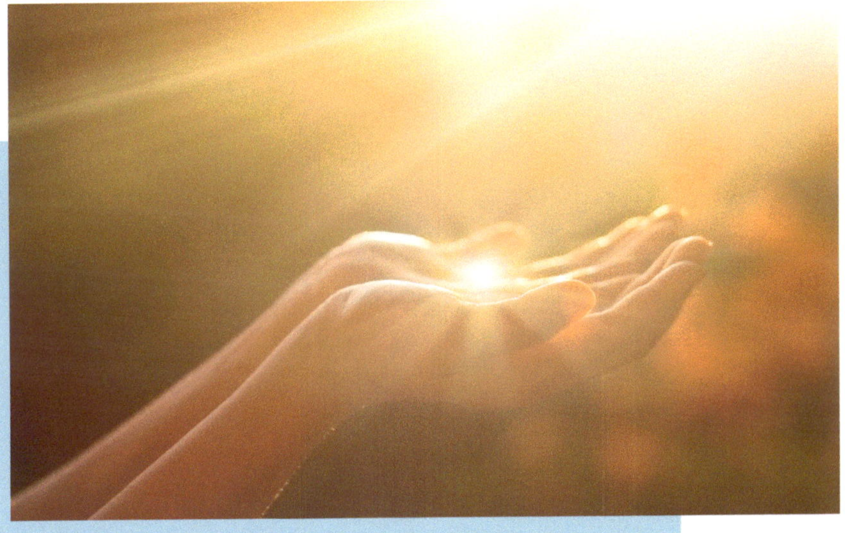

GIVE IT TO GOD

I never would have survived if I didn't have God in my life, I kid you not. If you aren't a God-lover, I won't be mad if you skip this part, but I can't skip it.

I would sit with my child, hear them, breathe with them. When they were able to breathe on their own, I would ask if I could leave. I would kiss them on the head, and tell them to come and wake me for any reason.

Then I would literally pray "God, I have to sleep. Please keep my baby alive tonight." And I would go to sleep.

I slept well. Night was the only respite from long, difficult, painful days.

But God took over for me while I slept. When I woke each morning, my heart halted as I entered their room, my breath stilled, fear threatened. But each morning they were alive. My heart resumed beating and breath returned to my lungs.

There are things we are not able to do on our own and we know it. We want to control things, but control is not always ours to have. We must give it over, and in doing that, if we are able to trust, we may find some peace.

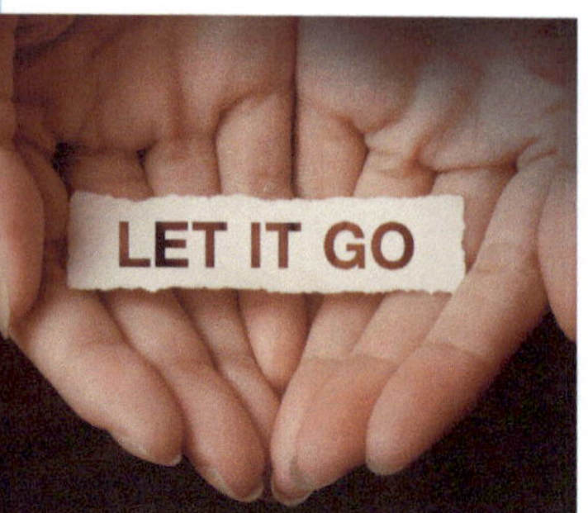

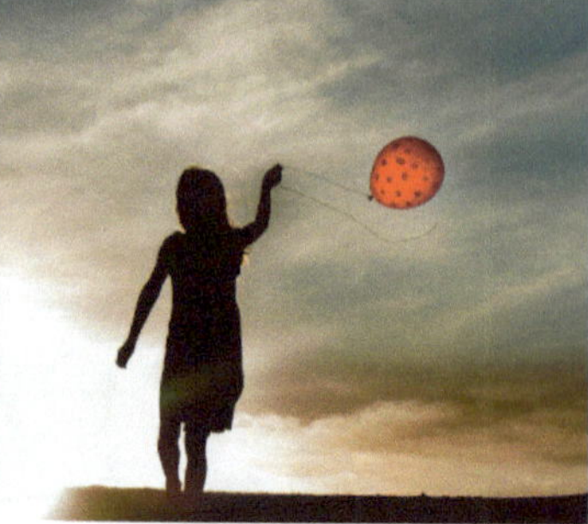

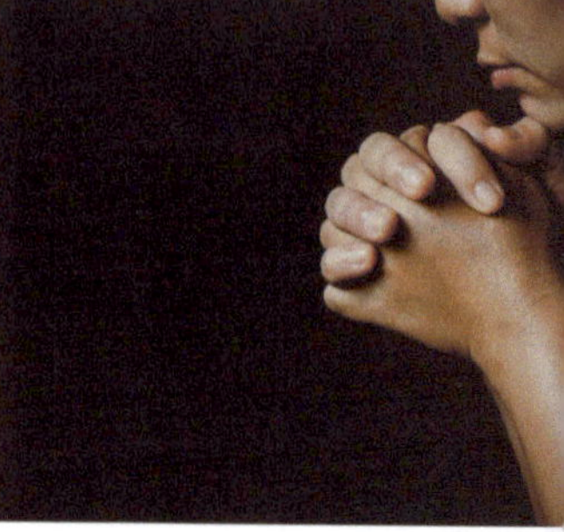

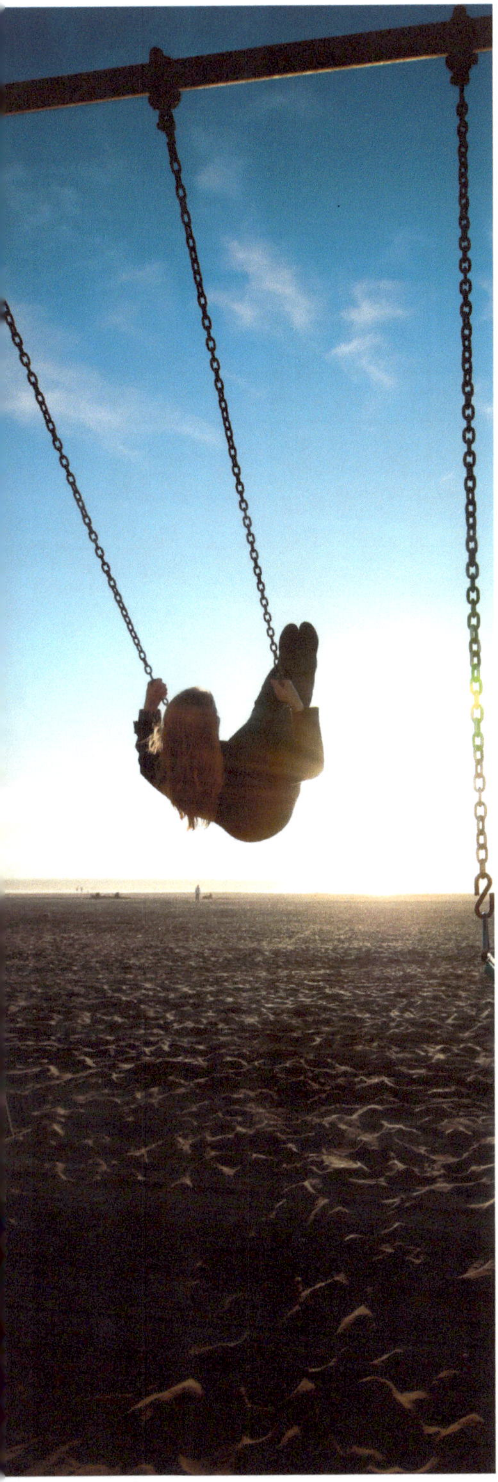

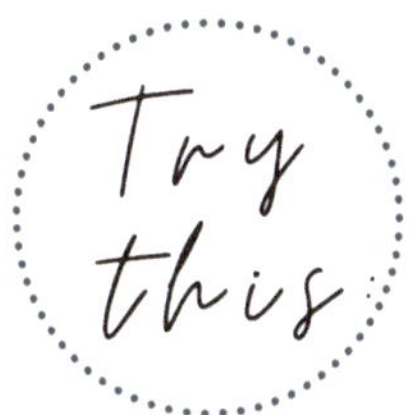

Give it to God and go to sleep

Let go and Let God...

Are these ideas that you haven't been using?

What do you need to let go of?

What has been so heavy on your mind that you are struggling with it every day?

Fear of being sick? Death? Isolation? That would make sense, wouldn't it?

Decide on one thing that you would like to release. Then choose one of the following activities.

- Write it on the sidewalk in chalk and spray it off with the hose.

- Write it on a piece of paper and burn it, (safely)

- Write it in sand on a beach and watch the waves wash it away.

- Write it on a leaf in Sharpie and watch it blow away in the wind.

- Open your hands and imagine God taking it from you.

No matter what you choose, be intentional about releasing that heavy thing. Breathe. Let it go. Give it to God.

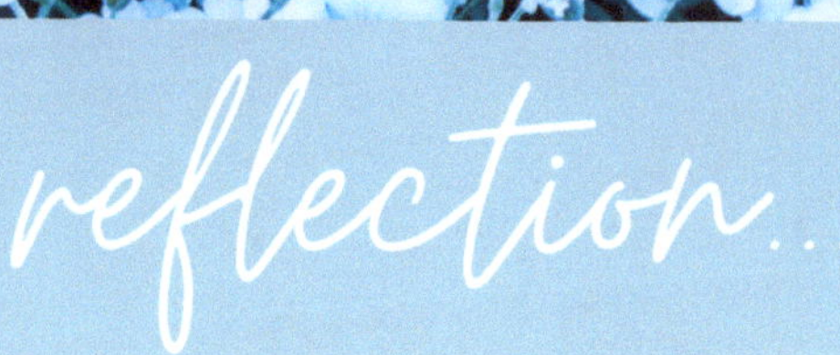

What I tried: _______________________________

How I felt before the exercise:
____
____
____

How I felt afterward:
____
____
____

What I liked about it:
____
____
____

What I didn't like about it:
____
____
____

Additional thoughts:
____
____

Would I try it again?_______________________________________

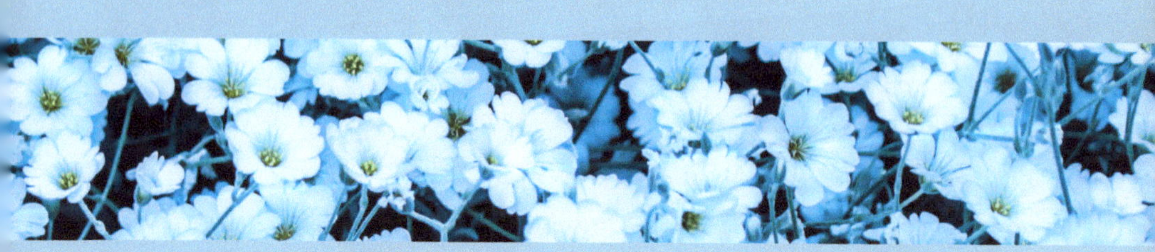

Notes

NINE:
FIND THE GOOD

"Find the good. It's all around you. Find it,
showcase it, and you'll start believing in it."
-Unknown

Raise your hand if you've heard of a gratitude journal. Okay, so I know nobody raised their hand, but I also know that all of you have heard of a gratitude journal. It's not a new concept, but it doesn't seem to go away- do you know why? Because it works. When you are intentional about finding the good things in your life, you see more of them. You are literally re-wiring your brain to see positives instead of negatives. Your brain will look for confirmation that things are good- instead of bad. It really really works.

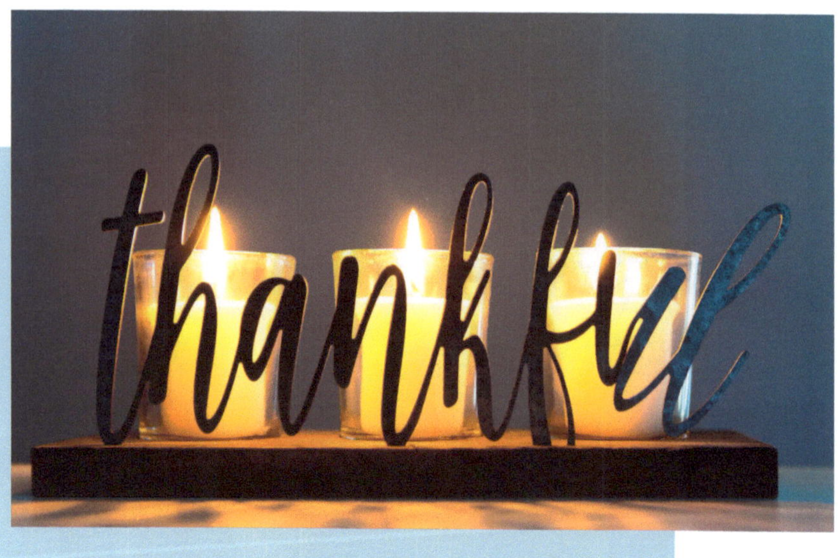

FIND THE GOOD

I heard a theory on mindset once. I have no idea where I heard it, but credit does not go to me. The idea is that in our minds we have two rooms. One room is hung with all of the negative stuff we've encountered in our lives, all of the things that annoy us, people who have treated us badly, disappointments we've endured, The other room is wall to wall papered with things that bring us joy. Pictures of people that we love, pets, beautiful places, favourite foods, good smells, amazing memories. The rooms are right next door to one another, but we cannot be in both rooms at the same time.

Which room are you in? Sometimes we've been in a negative headspace for so long we forget that right next door is a room of wonderful, so here's your reminder. Figure out which room you're in, and then decide which room you *want* to be in. I'm hoping you'll pick the joyful one, and plant yourself there. Settle in, let yourself flourish. Watch the room fill with more and more good things. You might be surprised if it starts to flow over into the negative room, changing the vibe altogether.

If you find yourself having a bad day, or going over a conversation in your head a bunch of times because someone really made you mad... get out of that room! Go next door. It's so close and makes all the difference.

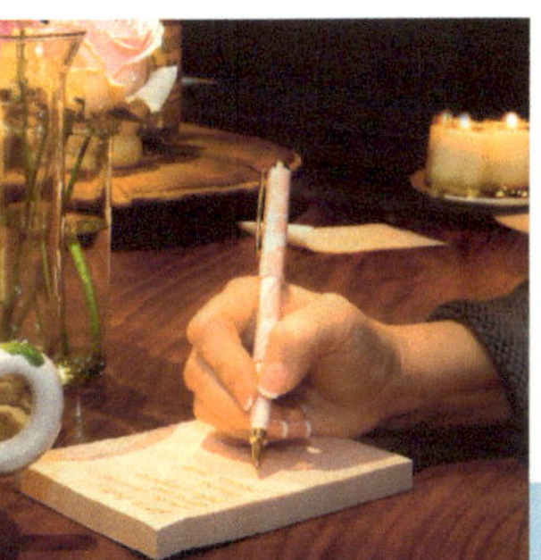
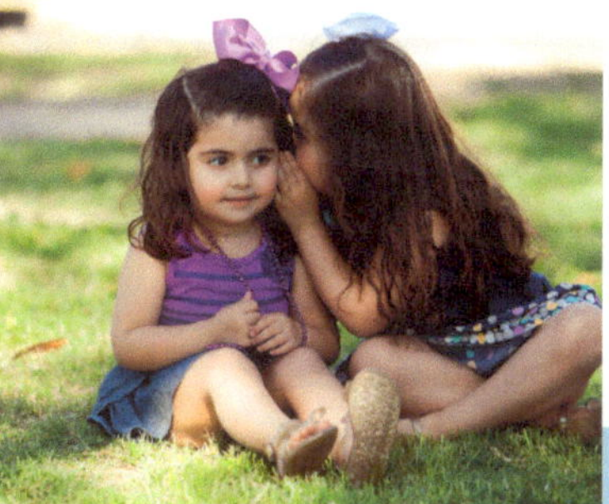
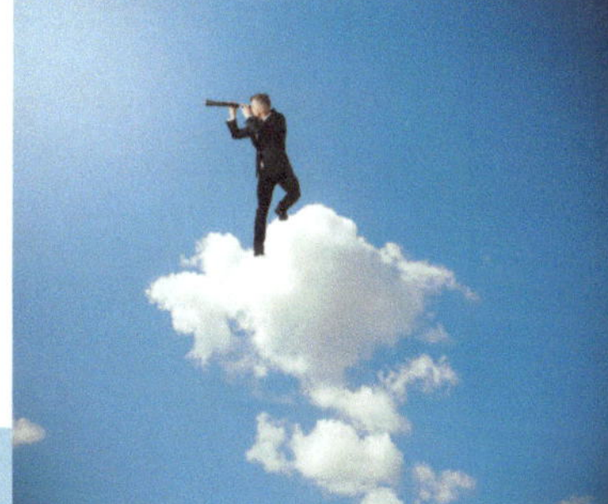

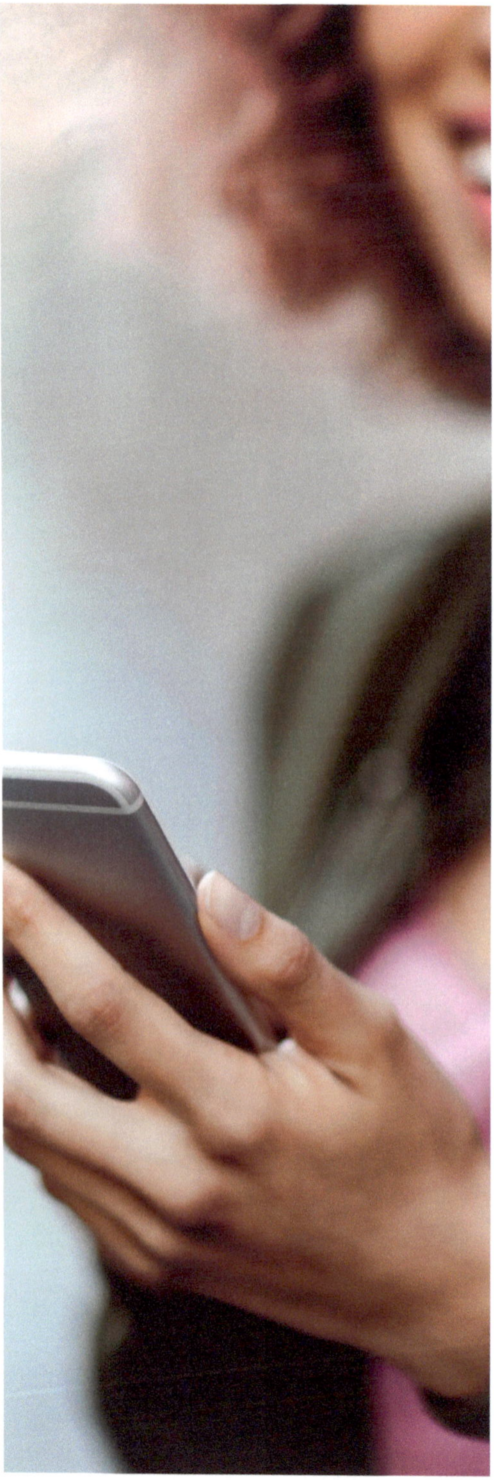

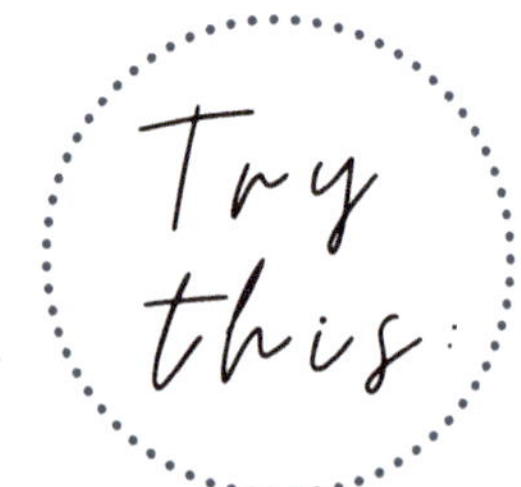

Try this:

Every morning or every evening send a text to someone thanking them for something. It could be something specific, like "Thanks for bringing our garbage can back when the wind blew it down the street. You are a great neighbour." It might be something a little more personal, "Thanks for always being there for me, you always make me feel loved and special."

Go grab a notebook. (If you're like me, go spend an hour or two looking at the new ones before choosing just the perfect one for this). Then sit down and write those 3 things you're thankful for. Repeat daily. As you write them, imagine you are pasting them up on the wall of your joy-filled room.

Some days you might have to work a little harder to find the good, but it's always a treasure worth hunting for.

Think about the negative room. Are there any things in there that you could let go of? Things that you don't need anymore? That aren't serving you? Feel free to use the practices of the last step (letting go) to let some of these go.

Share with others something you are thankful for. Talk about it in conversation with co-workers, post about it on Facebook or Instagram, tell your children. Make gratitude a part of your everyday life.

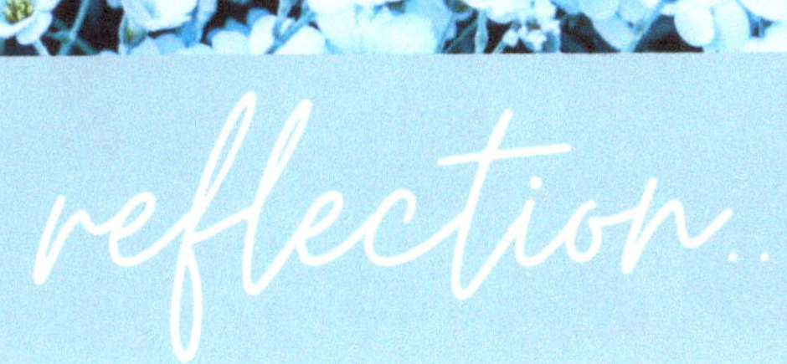

What I tried: ____

How I felt before the exercise: _______________________________
____
____

How I felt afterward: ____
____
____

What I liked about it: ____
____
____

What I didn't like about it: ___________________________________
____
____

Additional thoughts: ____
____

Would I try it again? _______________________________________

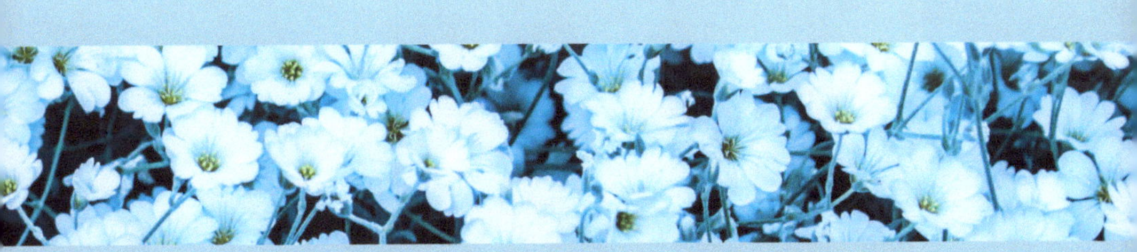

Notes

TEN: SMILE

10

"Smile, smile, smile at your mind as often as possible. Your smiling will considerably reduce your mind's tearing tension."
-Sri Chinmoy

Did you know that smiling makes you feel better? I learned this years ago, and made my kids smile at me on the way out the door to school, every day. It didn't even matter if it was a "fake" smile. Why? Because science. When our face uses those smile muscles, our brain receives a signal that says we're happy, and releases a bunch of beautiful buzzing endorphins, which then make us actually happy! How amazing is that? I read that one smile makes your brain as happy as 2000 chocolate bars! That's a lot of happy. Smiling reduces blood pressure and stress hormones too. It's all-over good for us. Try it right now. Happy or not, make that face smile, and see what you notice.

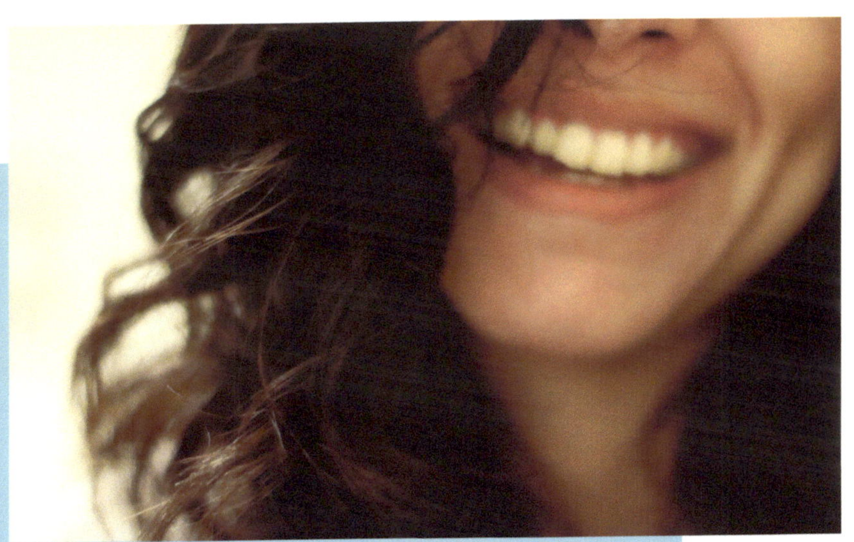

SMILE

"It only takes a split second to smile and forget, yet to someone that needed it, it can last a lifetime." — Steve Maraboli

Not only does smiling make you feel better- it also makes other people feel better! Smiles are contagious.

For years I've been playing what I call "The Smile Game". It is most effective in a big city where everyone is in a hurry. I walk down the mall making eye contact with strangers and smiling at them. Most people do a double take, and then end up smiling right back. I love how startled they are that someone is actually smiling right at them.

Humans are wired to mimic the expressions of those around us in order to express empathy. We reflect sadness when someone is sad, and happiness when they are happy (ie. smile when they do).

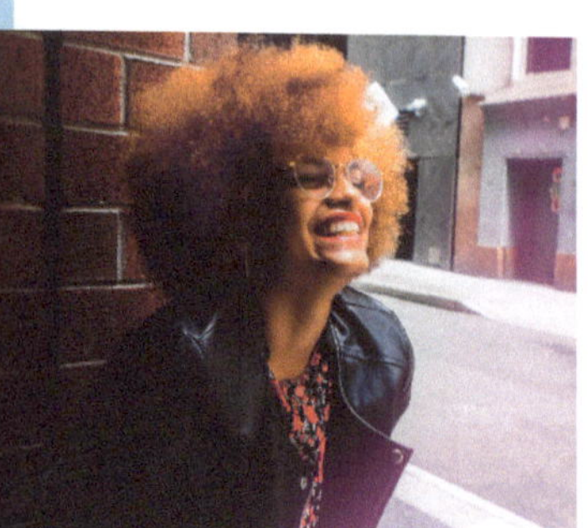 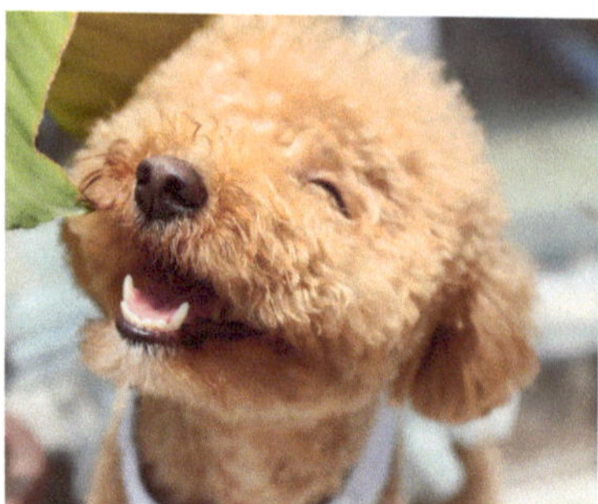 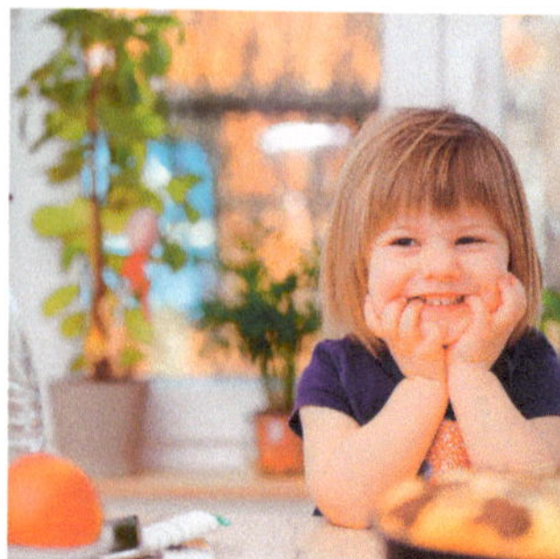

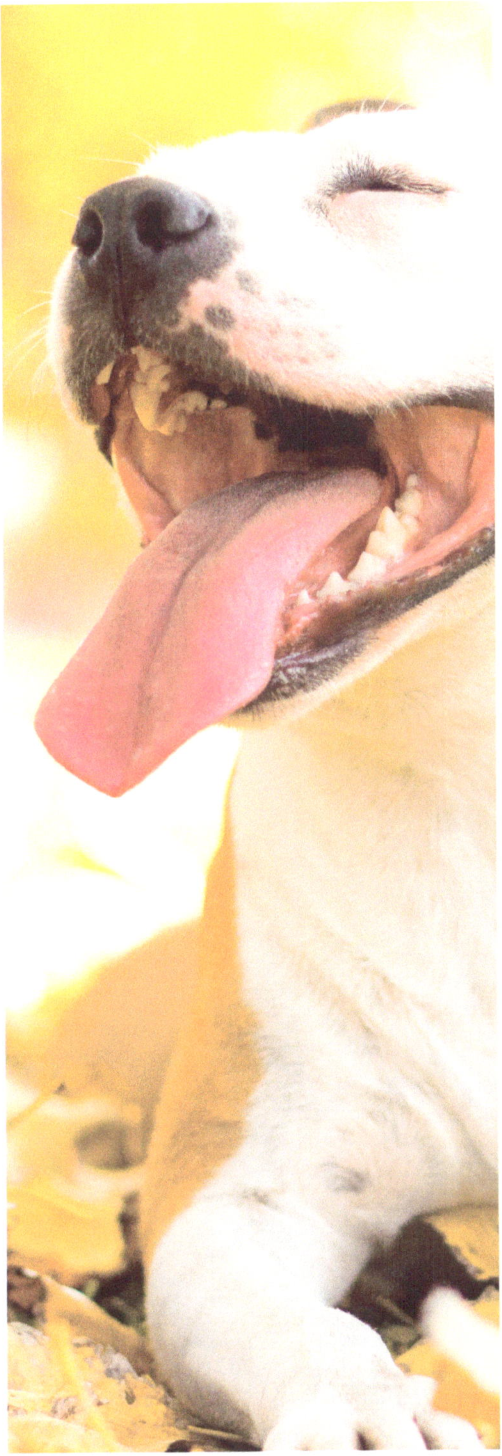

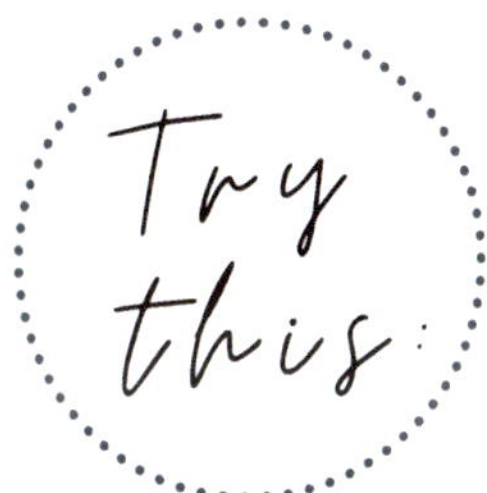

Smile every time you think about it. Notice your mood elevate. Notice the way you think about things more positively. Notice how gratitude sneaks into your heart.

Try "The Smile Game". Find a busy place, make eye contact with others, and see if they smile back. Remember that sometimes they may smile after they've already passed you. People are not used to eye contact or physical communication like smiles. Most have their faces buried in cell phones, completely unaware of the people around them.

Give out smiles like gifts. Just acknowledging someone can make their whole day.

Note: Some people hate their smile and most people think they look better when they're not smiling. You'll often see profile pictures of people with a straight face, and wonder why they don't smile. That's why. But- most of the time, if given a choice of pictures (one smiling and one not) everyone other than the pictured individual will choose the smiling one. Why? Because smiles are contagious. Seeing even a picture of someone we care about smiling brings a smile to our face too, making us feel all those wonderful happy feelings.

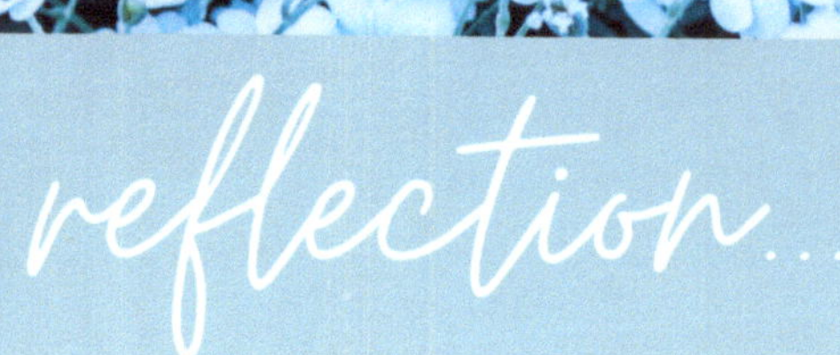

What I tried: ____

How I felt before the exercise: _______________________________

____

____

How I felt afterward: ____

____

____

What I liked about it: ____

____

____

What I didn't like about it: __________________________________

____

____

Additional thoughts: ____

____

Would I try it again? ______________________________________

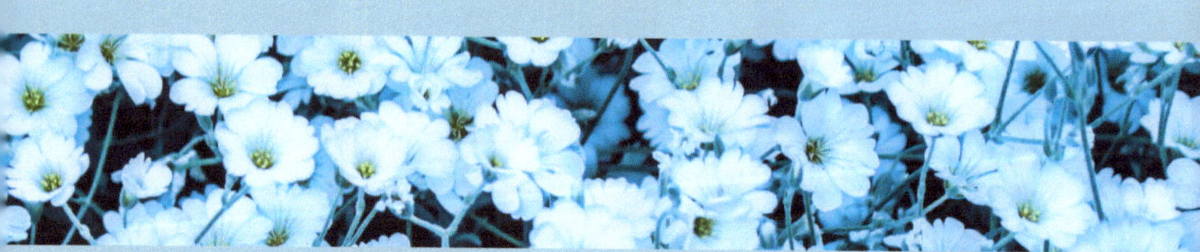

Notes

Conclusion...

So... did you try? What did you find the most helpful? What didn't help at all? Did you recognize yourself anywhere in the reading? What could you share with someone else?

Your very existence is to be celebrated. The world can seem so big, so dark, so scary and unfair. And you have survived. Well done.

In the days to come, I pray that you will use these skills on such a regular basis that you don't even notice. That you will breathe easy, look on the bright side, and rest when you need to. That you will notice your impact on the world, and will create something beautiful with the time you've been given. Make connections, ground yourself , pray, and get away.

Be blessed, my friends,

You certainly are a blessing.

Charlaine

> *"Take care of you, because that's who you'll be spending the rest of your life with."*

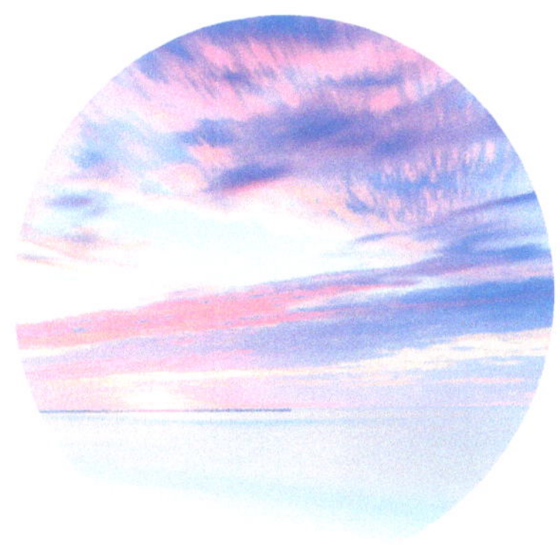

If you enjoyed this book, please consider
leaving a review on

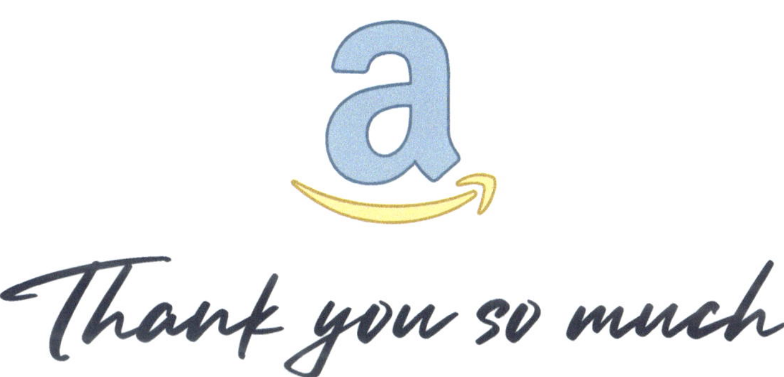

Thank you so much